GENES, DREAMS AND REALITIES

GENES DREAMS AND REALITIES

SIR MACFARLANE BURNET

MTP

Medical and Technical Publishing Co Ltd
Chiltern House, Oxford Road
Aylesbury, Bucks

Published in Great Britain
in 1971 by

MTP

Medical and Technical Publishing Co Ltd
Chiltern House, Oxford Road
Aylesbury, Bucks

ISBN-13: 978-94-011-7134-2   e-ISBN-13: 978-94-011-7132-8
DOI: 10.1007/978-94-011-7132-8

CONTENTS

1

INTRODUCTION TO GENES

The stimulus to write this book came from a suggestion that too much sensational material was being written about the future significance for medicine of discoveries in molecular biology, and that it was desirable that someone with my sort of background should attempt a popularly written but critical account of how in the light of current research and opinion the future technical patterns of preventive and curative medicine may develop. It was also mentioned that a few years ago I gained some short-lasting notoriety by suggesting that molecular biology, far from promising brave new achievements in medicine, might release some new and nasty problems on a world which has already more than it can cope with. Could I produce a balanced account of where modern biological science has brought us and how that knowledge can be applied in the future to matters bearing directly on the quality of human life? Are we going to see 'genetic engineering' applied to the cure of genetic disease or to the conscious production of a race of supermen? Will we ever live in health for three hundred years or stretch our lives over even longer periods by spending a century every now and then deep-frozen but still viable? Or will the future, as far as medicine and human genetics are concerned, be very like the present but with a progressively wider spread of present potential benefits over the world's populations? Perhaps the most important thing to be gained from trying to answer such questions is the opportunity it gives to clarify one's ideas about what in the 1970s medical research has as its main objectives.

Research in the fields relevant to medicine has expanded continuously since the beginning of this century and has won for itself a high level of public appreciation. But its approach, the type of problems being studied, and the form taken by its discoveries have been changing progressively. It is no longer relevant to speak of penicillin and the other wonder drugs of the 1940s and 1950s as a sufficient answer. One of the themes which will run through this book is that medicine in the broad sense is concerned almost with two different universes. Disease and disability may result from the impact of the environment or they may be generated intrinsically to the body. Intrinsic disease broadly results from genetic error. Either in the body as a whole or in individual cells, genes are missing or not functioning as they should.

As it has developed, my objective in writing this book has become to present from a broad biological and human standpoint the main features of those diseases, disabilities, or harmless anomalies that are directly related to fault within the body's complement of genes. Only with a background of this natural history of genetic and somatic genetic disease is it legitimate to attempt to predict how far current or foreseeable discoveries will allow us to handle what have become in the last thirty years the main group of conditions for which men and women seek relief in the consulting rooms and hospitals of the Western world.

Perhaps the first thing needed is to warn the reader that modern medicine and medical science is by no means such a triumphal march toward perpetual health and well-being as popular accounts of what is going on in the research laboratories might lead the simple-minded to picture. It will become necessary to explain why pneumonia and tonsillitis are easily cured, why diphtheria and polio have vanished, yet cancer in general, coronary thrombosis, and mental disease are more prevalent and not very much more effectively treated than they were. It has been exciting to watch the expectation of life at birth in almost all affluent Western countries creep up to something like 74 for women and 68 for men in the early 1960s. But it has stayed almost the same since then. It is always easier to produce an interesting account of the successes of medicine than to write entertainingly of things hard to understand and harder to change which continue to ensure that all men die.

Let me try to sketch the bare essentials of the picture of medical science as it presents in 1970. Since the days of Pasteur and Lister, science and common sense have found their most effective application to medicine by concentrating on those causes of disease that clearly come from without. By dealing with infectious disease, by rationalizing nutrition, and providing safe food and water, and by applying well-tested methods of resuscitation and surgery to the casualties of war and the roads, countless lives have been saved and a new security given to human existence. Medical research was not wholly responsible but it was the core of the matter and it was natural that its achievements should attract the admiration and goodwill of the world. In the years between roughly 1930 and 1955 the discoveries seemed to come thick and fast and the mass media developed to make them more widely known than before. The proclamation of exciting discoveries continues unabated and it is not easy to recognize that the character of the discoveries has changed. Most people, even most doctors, seem to be waiting hopefully for a great set of new cures and new preventive procedures. But a discovery made once is never made again and it may be that most of the discoveries needed for practical medicine have been made.

The success of, and the prestige attaching to medical research came in dealing with what I have come to speak of as the impact of the environment. Physical injury, infection, and malnutrition; these are the types of disability that we have learnt to understand by the systematic use of the scientific method in the laboratory. Many types of infectious disease can be prevented and almost all serious types can be effectively treated if the right methods can be applied early enough. Malnutrition should no longer exist anywhere in the world. No wounded soldier or road victim should die if the resuscitation team arrives before irremediable damage is done. What remains to be prevented and cured has a different set of origins. Broadly speaking, the conditions whose control eludes us have a genetic or a somatic genetic background against which the onset of deterioration can be accelerated by self-indulgence or misfortune.

This book is primarily concerned with the significance of 'genes' for the medical problems that continue almost unabated despite our success in dealing with the 'environmental' diseases. I am going to assume that any one reading this book will have a reasonable background of interest in biology even though he has forgotten every vestige of detail about Mendel's laws or what the letters DNA stand for.

Everyone has a working knowledge of the meaning of the word 'gene' and I shall use it frequently, though I am very much aware that it is an extremely difficult word to define satisfactorily. Similarly, DNA, which stands for deoxyribonucleic acid, has become almost common coin in English with very much the same connotation as gene. Again, an accurate definition of DNA means nothing to the person who has no knowledge of organic chemistry. I want to avoid writing anything like the first chapter of an elementary textbook of genetics, but I do want to clarify as quickly as possible the implications of genetics for human disease at both of what one calls the germinal and somatic levels.

Perhaps it may be helpful to start with a greatly oversimplified statement of modern genetic theory. According to this, there is present in the nucleus of the fertilized egg cell from which a new human being develops, all the information—the blueprints and specifications as it were—that is needed to determine the form and function of the future infant, child, and adult. The information is stored in the chemical structure of the long threads of DNA which are the chief constituent of the visible chromosomes of the nucleus. A gene, physically speaking, is a segment of DNA carrying a unit of information, such as how to make a certain protein. The word is, however, used more often in genetics for a useful concept that has been developed for explaining in terms of discrete units, the inheritable differences between people or between plants and animals of the same species.

As a more practical introduction to the topic and as a road to defining 'gene', 'germinal', and 'somatic', I believe that there is much to be gained by talking about albinos in a brown-skinned people.

GENES IN THE TROBRIAND ISLANDERS

Three or four years ago I spent one of the most fascinating weekends I have ever experienced on Kirawina the largest of the Trobriand Islands north-east of New Guinea. Three of us, all interested in medical research and one very much of an anthropologist, had heard that there was an unusually high proportion of albinos amongst Trobriand Islanders. The Government medical officer on the island was interested in the condition and was happy to offer us hospitality and transport around the villages. In due course we saw five of the twelve albinos he knew of.

Kirawina is a large coral island 50 miles long with a population of about 10,000. It lies right in the track of Pacific migrations and there are obviously both Polynesian and Melanesian genes in the population. These were the people about whom Malinowski wrote his *Sex in Savage Society*. Since then the Pacific war and the

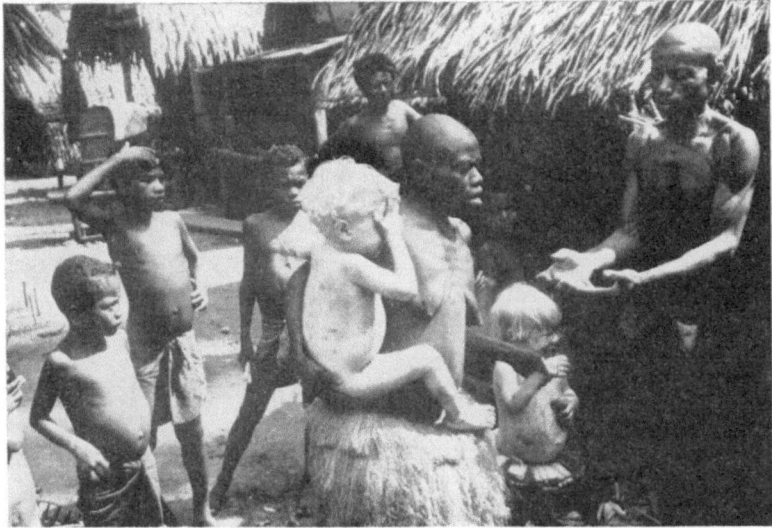

FIG. 1. Two albino children of the brown-skinned Trobriand Islanders of mixed Indonesian/Polynesian stock. The children show inflamed areas of skin but no pigmented patches.

establishment of two American airstrips on Kirawina have intervened, but superficially at least the people have retained much of their old way of life and of their cheerful temperament. The highest knoll on the island is only 30 ft above sea level and the wartime jeep tracks are still in good order. To go in a Land-Rover from one village to another with a guide who was interested in both medical and social aspects of his 'practice' was sheer joy.

But the albinos then, as now, were our business. We went first to see a family with two albino children, one an infant in arms the other 3 years old. The parents both had normal brown skins and the two earlier children were also brown. What interested us particularly was that both children were 'clean skins' with no brown patches or spots. Like all albinos they could not bear bright sunlight and hid their faces when brought out to be photographed.

Albinism is a typical genetic abnormality due to a recessive gene which shows what we call typical Mendelian behaviour. Human chromosomes are in pairs, one from the mother, one from the father; the genes in each chromosome correspond but are not necessarily identical. If there is a pair of genes both normal which

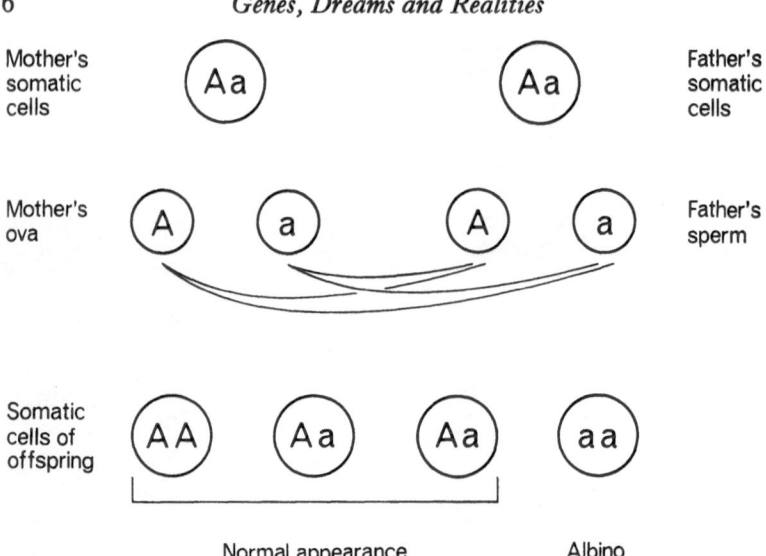

Mother's somatic cells — Aa

Father's somatic cells — Aa

Mother's ova — A   a

Father's sperm — A   a

Somatic cells of offspring — AA   Aa   Aa   aa

Normal appearance   Albino

FIG. 2. Albinism as a recessive genetic trait.

we call AA the individual has the normal brown skin colour. But an abnormal gene a can arise by mutation of A and when an individual has two abnormal genes aa, he is born an albino. Any one with one of each type Aa is brown, and quite indistinguishable from any one else. This is the reason for saying that a is recessive to A. In a tropical country albinos usually die young and, though in the Trobriands they are accepted fully and well cared for, they are subject to a taboo on marriage. It follows that the marriages which produce albinos (aa) are always between an Aa man and an Aa woman. Everyone knows the equation $Aa \times Aa$ gives $1AA$: $2Aa : 1aa$, so with a very little arithmetic it appears that with a ratio of albinos to normals around $1 : 1,000$ about 1 person in every 16 must be an Aa carrier of the gene for albinism. Most of the genetic diseases we find in European communities have the same type of recessive behaviour with, on the average, only 1 in 4 of the offspring of $Aa \times Aa$ marriages showing the disease.

Before leaving this matter of numbers, it may be good for the reader if I interpolate an experience with albinos on the New Guinea mainland. At Madang the MO knew of 'a whole family of albinos' and arranged for them all to be available on a Sunday morning to be photographed. The photograph shows two dark-

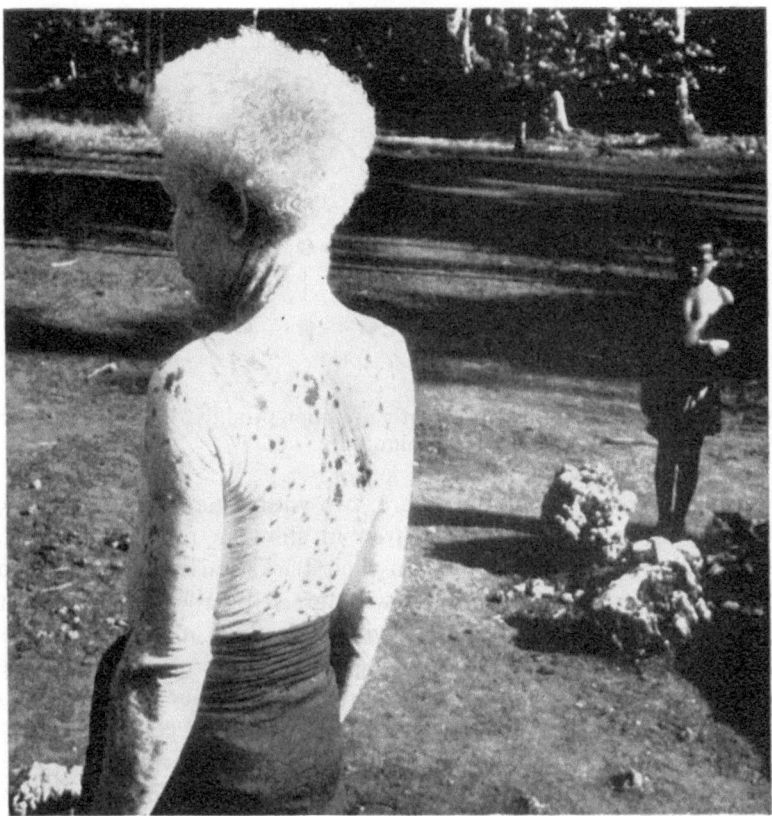

F IG. 3. Another Trobriand Islander albino. A boy of about 17 showing brown irregular patches of pigmentation on his back and arms.

skinned parents and seven children, two brown and five albinos. If the ratio had been in the opposite direction I should have used the slide for any lecture on human genetics that I shall ever give. As it is I tell myself that a ratio that 'should' be 1:3 will on statistical principles appear as 5:2 once in 1,700 families; or that this family must have had more than one gene capable of producing or assisting to produce albinism. It is rather characteristic of biological generalizations to come up against difficulties of this sort—the finding that does not fit but is too rare to allow it to be properly studied.

The Trobriand albinos have, however, another lesson to teach

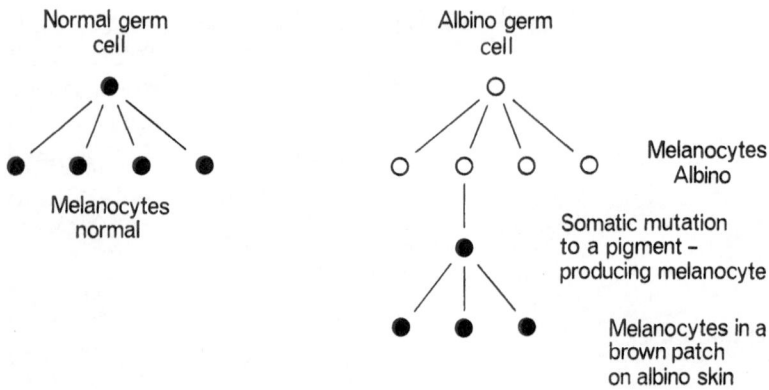

FIG. 4. An example of how somatic mutation produces brown patches on albino skin.

us. The three adult albinos there, two young men and a girl of 15 or 16, differed from the children in showing numerous brown spots and irregular patches, on their backs particularly but also on other parts of the body. It was agreed by their relatives that they, like all albinos, were born with clean skins and that the spots developed and enlarged as they grew older. Some of the spots looked much like a mole on a European skin but most of them were quite different, looking like an irregular frayed-out patch of melanesian pigmentation rather than a mole. Some were pigmented nodules which looked as if they might develop into one or other of the forms of skin cancer that in the tropics are unduly common in Europeans (basal cell carcinoma and malignant melanoma).

Those spots and patches were the result of *somatic* mutation. As a result of the germinal mutation from A to a and the occurrence in the albino of the two recessive genes aa some phase of the process by which the brown pigment, melanin, is synthesized in the melanocyte cells of the skin and elsewhere is blocked. The melanocytes are there but they do not make pigment. Any one who has watched a red-headed small boy develop freckles has seen an object lesson in how a melanocyte that makes more pigment than normal has the capacity to produce descendant melanocytes which can overgrow unchanged ones and produce a freckle. In the Trobriand albinos the inactive melanocytes are subject to mutation probably in part due to their absence of shielding from sunlight.

Amongst the mutations are some which either reverse the original germinal mutation to *A* or more likely induce a different type of genetic change which allows the blocked process to be circumvented, some form of metabolic bypass develops which again allows melanin to be produced by one somatic cell and its descendants. This gives them also the capacity to prosper and to grow and occupy new territory till they produce the visible spots with many thousands of pigmented melanocytes in each.

I have used this example of genetic disease or abnormality as it occurs in the germ-cell line—the sort of conditions to which we normally restrict the term, genetic disease—because of the ease with which the analogous somatic genetic changes, either in freckles or in the brown spots of Trobriand albinos can be recognized. I shall have much to say about somatic mutation and analogous matters and these examples give the opportunity to make an important point. A freckle is circular because it arises from a single cell whose descendants must proliferate at the expense of normal melanocytes if it is going to produce a visible freckle. All mutations are rare events involving a single cell whether in germ cells or somatic cells, and, by rare, we mean something of the order of one in a million or less. It is both obvious and crucial to the understanding of the effects of somatic mutation that any change that involves only one cell in a million will be of no significance whatever unless it has an opportunity to proliferate very considerably and provide a large population of descendant cells, all exhibiting the mutant character.

FLEECE MOSAICS IN SHEEP

This same principle of the need for cell proliferation to magnify the effect of somatic mutation is beautifully illustrated in another example from my own part of the world. It concerns fleece mosaics in Australian sheep. The standard merino and crossbred sheep bred in Australia have dense fleece each fibre of which has a wavy configuration, its crimp, which gives the characteristic appearance to the fleece on the sheep's back and allows the fleece to hang together after it has been shorn. Since the wool is the commercially important part of the sheep, any abnormalities are noticed immediately. Amongst such abnormalities which usually lead to the prompt slaughter of the lamb showing them, was the appearance

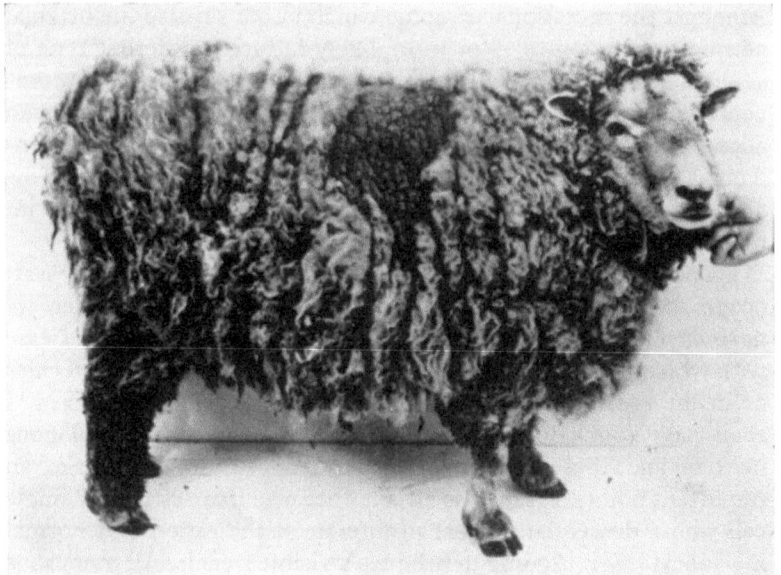

FIG. 5. An example of fleece mosaic. A sheep with 50 per cent of body area with long fleece (Fraser and Short, *Aust. J. Biol. Sci.* **2** (1958), 200).

of substantial patches of long loosely crimped wool contrasting with the normal firm fleece on the rest of the animal. Fraser and Short in the 1950s became interested in these sheep and arranged for an extensive survey of Australian flocks. They believe that in fact they obtained virtually all the animals showing any considerable degree of this long fleece mosaic condition, in some 20 million sheep. It was something no sheepman could miss and there was a good liaison between the Commonwealth Scientific and Industrial Research Organization (CSIRO) and the wool growers.

The fascinating feature of the results when 22 mosaic sheep were obtained and examined was that if the sheep were divided into groups according to the proportion of wool in the long form, the number in each group was inversely proportional to the area of skin involved. There was 1 sheep with almost exactly 50 per cent of its skin area involved, 3 with about 25 per cent, 4 around 10 or 12 per cent, and increasing numbers with lesser degrees. Fraser and Short deduced that they were dealing with one particular

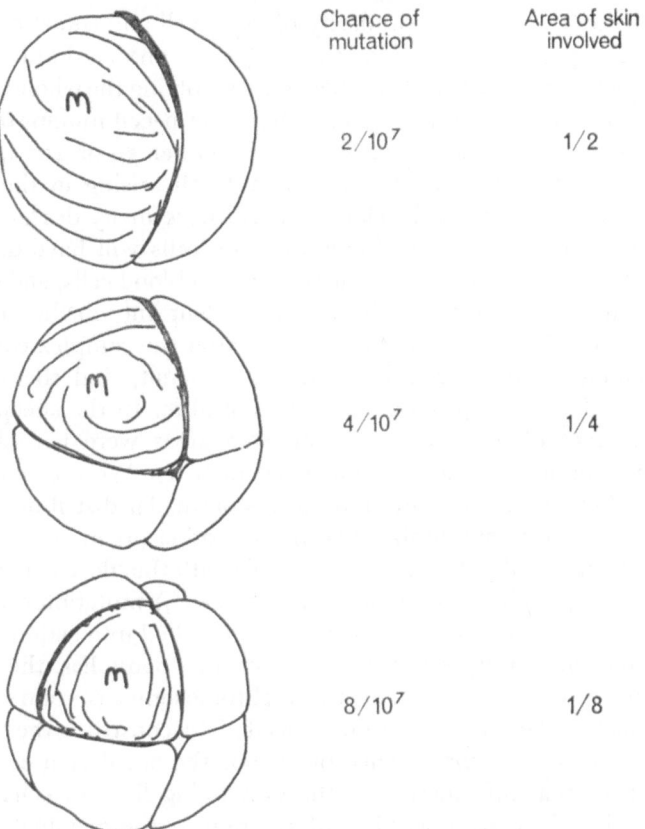

	Chance of mutation	Area of skin involved
	$2/10^7$	$1/2$
	$4/10^7$	$1/4$
	$8/10^7$	$1/8$

FIG. 6. The origin of fleece mosaics in sheep. The diagram shows the effects of somatic mutation taking place early in the history of the fertilized ovum. With only one cell (M) mutating, the proportion of descendant cells involved will diminish the later mutation occurs, but examples of mutation will be more frequent.

type of somatic mutation which might occur at any period of embryonic development and was just as likely to occur during the lifetime of any one cell as of any other. If it occurred to involve one of the two cells from the first division of the fertilized ovum, 50 per cent of the fleece would be involved but, if a cell in the sixteen-cell stage were involved, only 5 or 6 per cent would be affected.

This has some important implications. The first is the way it

establishes the essential similarity of germ cell and somatic mutations. No germ-cell mutation of this type was observed but several
examples of mutant fleece of other types involving the whole animal
were found and one cannot doubt that a germ-cell mutant of long
fleece type would have been found, if another 50 or 100 million
sheep had been looked at! Any mutant cell arising in the early
stages of the embryo's development will have many descendants,
all carrying the mutation. Some of those cells will have descendants that are muscle cells, some that are red blood cells, and so on.
The mutation, however, will become evident only in the descendants of the original mutant cell which, after the complex comings
and goings of differentiation and development, find themselves
responsible for the production of a wool fibre. In the sheep with
50 per cent of long fleece the affected areas were lens-shaped
regions running vertically from back to belly. We are not concerned here with why they showed this particular distribution but
it is important to emphasize that in every other organ of the sheep
there would be about 50 per cent of cells with the 'fleece' mutation
without any evidence at all of their existence. A mutation can only
be recognized when the gene concerned is called into action for its
predetermined purpose. Every cell of the body has the same
number of chromosomes and those chromosomes contain all the
information, all the 'blueprints', needed to construct the whole
body. But it is of the essence of all but the smallest unicellular
organisms that information in the developing lines of cells from
the fertilized ovum onward—'information in the genome' is the
compact way of saying it—is expressed only in those cells where
it can be used for the proper needs of the organism.

Neither of the examples of albinism or fleece mosaics in sheep
is directly concerned with human disease in the ordinary sense.
I believe, however, that they do give some important insight into
the problems of medicine that are now becoming important and
will make the concept of somatic mutation in its medical implications easier to understand. Those two examples also serve to
underline some other aspects of genetics and bodily development.

The first is the marvellous and intimidating complexity of the
mechanism of life. I think that only those who have experienced
the extraordinary amount of information and instruction which
must be fed into a computer to allow it to do something relatively
simple like translating a Russian technical article into English can

realize the inconceivable subtlety of the process by which in every nucleus of the body there are the same molecular memory stores and operational instructions as those which allow the fertilized ovum to grow to a man. The sheep story shows how what seems a completely trivial bit of information is carried through hundreds of cell generations till it reaches the only point where it can be expressed. Sheep-breeders will tell you that they are breeding for this, that, or the other character of fleece which influences its field of use and its market value. Each is somehow represented in the genome. I am professionally interested in the fine structure and function of the cell surface in relation to immunology. Here it seems that there is an inconceivable complexity of direct and indirect genetic information brought to bear at the right time and according to the needs of the particular cell type. That information must have a molecular basis and molecular biology has in broad terms told us what that basis is. I shall discuss it in the next chapter. It is a fascinating story that made a bestseller of *The Double Helix* but it is liable to give a totally wrong idea of simplicity in living function.

MUTABILITY UNLIMITED

The appearance of spots on albino skin which, like the freckles on some small boys' faces, may be of half a dozen different sorts, raises another point which has already been mentioned but may be elaborated in a somewhat different fashion. We can recognize the existence of a mutant only when conditions are such as allow it a proliferative advantage over its unchanged fellows. With pigment cells in the skin there is not much one can do except to observe what nature allows to happen but with bacteria it is different.

Much of modern genetics and biochemistry has come from work on common, easily grown bacteria, especially the one we all call *Escherichia coli*. As one geneticist put it, 'It has almost become an article of faith that if it happens in *E. coli*, it will also happen in an elephant.' Mutations take place in bacteria probably at much the same rate as they do in melanocytes and in both cases you get more if you expose them to ultra-violet light. Bacteria, however, have one great advantage for experimental work. If the investigator is looking for any particular type of mutant he can usually arrange the situation so that the mutant he is interested in will grow while unmutated forms will not. The simplest possible example is when a penicillin-resistant mutant is wanted. All that is needed is to put enough penicillin into the plate of nutrient agar (on which bacterial colonies are counted) to prevent growth of the particular microbe being studied. Then the plate is spread with, say, 10 million bacteria from a pure culture and incubated. Only ten colonies may develop from the whole 10 million. The appropriate tests will usually show that the few million bacteria in such a colony are just like the parent colony in all respects except that they have become resistant to the killing effect of penicillin. There are dozens of more subtle ways of arranging for this or that mutant to have an advantage, and long experience allows us to generalize fairly confidently: that bacteria are subject to an enormous range of possible mutations and if there is the physical possibility of a mutation it will occur. With enough ingenuity it is usually possible to arrange conditions so that the mutant will proliferate and produce what we call a *clone* of the new type, i.e., a family of descendants successively 2, 4, 8, etc., while unmutated cells fail to multiply. This allows what is technically called isolating the mutant. All mutations, however, are rare and random, some rarer than others but for the most part occurring around one per million. Everything suggests that mutation in animal or human cells takes place in similar rare, random, and diverse fashion. Here, however, the mutation itself must provide the opportunity for proliferation that will allow the mutant to be recognized.

These characteristics of genetic phenomena—that changes are rare, random, and very diverse and that, given the appropriate environment in which it has opportunity for selective survival, the rarest mutant can be grown to an unlimited amount—call for a special sort of logical and mathematical approach.

THE STOCHASTIC (RANDOM) APPROACH IN MEDICINE

For nearly fifteen years I have been preaching the importance of somatic genetic processes as the basis of some important types of human disease including cancer and of the corresponding conditions when they occur in domestic animals or some laboratory model. It is not a popular approach either to practising physicians or to scientists concerned with the laboratory investigation of such diseases. Their resistance to the idea is due in large part to the legitimate opinion of most experimental scientists that it is not helpful to ascribe a biological phenomenon to a process which cannot be produced to order in an experimental animal and studied in the laboratory. Equally potent probably is the less sophisticated commonsense view of layman and doctor that every illness, every recognizable clinical appearance in the patient has an identifiable cause. If the bacterium known as the pneumococcus produces pneumonia, a virus must produce cancer, and some mysterious chemical or another virus must produce auto-immune disease. As yet the concept of a stochastic as contrasted with a determinative approach to the understanding of disease has made relatively little progress in the medical schools. In the simplest possible terms there are some diseases whose incidence, when looked at from the point of view of the individual patient, falls wholly at random. But when one looks at a few thousand cases and sorts them out as to age and sex, a certain regularity emerges and depending on the particular disease, other regularities in relation to environmental factors will become visible. The incidence of cancer of the lung has the basically random character of any other cancer but this can be almost dominated by a characteristic relationship to intensity of cigarette smoking and modified by other factors such as life in urban or country areas. Random processes which only make sense when looked at statistically are found through almost the whole physical universe. As Schrodinger pointed out in *What is Life*, only molecules and crystals can on occasion have a persisting existence not perpetually subject to wholly random processes.

In the biological world, evolution is based on mutation, recombination, and the chances of survival; all random (stochastic) processes. The rules of evolution can be expressed mathematically only in terms of probabilities. Evolutionary change is concerned essentially with the processes by which the various possible 'genotypes' each with its own characteristic pattern of inheritance are distributed through the population being considered. Each type will have its own probability of surviving and having offspring, and that probability will differ according to environmental circumstances.

Any individual animal's good or bad fortune is an irrelevant statistic.

A doctor is trained to diagnose and treat the individual patient and in a sense to accept a certain responsibility when his patient fails to survive. At various times in my career I have, like many another medical philosopher, become deeply interested in graphs of specific age incidence of causes of death. There is a fascinating regularity about such curves, every one of which is made up of thousands of points representing a death of a human being at age x from disease y. For any individual who by his death comes into one of those curves, excuses will be made. It will be said that he was not treated early enough, that he had been under mental stress before he became ill or that there was some residual disability from the First World War or something quite different but equally factual and convincing. But the graph says without possibility of refutation that considered as a population the death-rate by ages was determined by stochastic regularities.

In concentrating, as I shall be, on intrinsic causes of disease there will be need to harp more than once on these differences between stochastic and determinative approaches. For the non-mathematical, like myself, the specific age incidence curve of reported disease or of death from a particular disease will remain the best approach to the understanding of how random factors are concerned in the incidence of disease and how they may be modified by both intrinsic and environmental factors. Several such graphs are used in later chapters.

Probably the prize that the public most longs to see won, is the discovery of the cause and cure of cancer. In 1957 I wrote a short series of articles on the biology of cancer and a brief article on the clonal selection theory of immunity. Both were based on a stochastic approach to somatic mutation in body cells. I was fortunate with the theory of immunity which by the end of the next ten years had been generally accepted as the basis on which modern theoretical ideas would be developed. This was primarily because during that time a whole set of new discoveries made sense on the clonal selection approach but not on the alternative that antigen could induce any cell to produce the corresponding antibody. It was particularly important that work on the disease, multiple myeloma, came to fruition during that decade. Myeloma can be regarded as a form of malignant, cancer-like proliferation of an antibody-producing cell giving rise to a very large clone of cells all producing an identical protein. This provided an easily understood model of how normal antibody-producing cells behaved.

The approach towards cancer that I adopted in 1957 was by no means original. Many writers had felt that the inheritable changes that are obviously present in cancer cells must arise by somatic mutation. The difficulty had been to understand why there were not many other kinds of somatic mutation as well as malignant ones. I fancy that I was saying something new when I emphasized that *only* when somatic mutation gave rise to a situation causing cellular proliferation would the fact that mutation had occurred, become manifest. This will need to be elaborated in the chapter on cancer but all that I want to say here is that those articles on cancer were written thirteen years ago. Since then, there has been furious activity in cancer research aimed mostly at proving that cancer was a virus disease or specifically due to various carcinogens including tobacco tar. I cannot see that any significant statements in that presentation of mine have been proved wrong over that thirteen years of research.

If the practical implications of research have not changed as a result of all the twenty-six years of laboratory work since the Second World War, then it must remain true that our methods of preventing or treating cancer must follow the lines that have been developed empirically in the past. These have been far from ineffective and the rules are basically simple. Prevent unnecessary exposure to agents which can increase the likelihood of mutation; remove or destroy all accessible groups of mutant cells which threaten life.

THE INFLUENCE OF IMMUNOLOGY

Whenever one writes about cancer or the degenerative diseases of the last third of life or about the process of ageing itself, immunological phenomena always seem to come into the picture. In the last twenty years I have had a good deal to do with the development of immunological theory and I may have a tendency to overplay its importance. Yet in a book on the general theme of genetic processes in relation to disease, somatic mutation and immune responses seem to demand almost equal consideration.

Immunity is usually thought of in the context of measles, polio, or diphtheria, something which protects one from infection that threatens from outside. Yet at the present time the growing edge of immunological research has moved quite away from its classical field of vaccination, serum treatment, diagnostic tests for past infection, and the like. Theory and practice are concerned much more with immune responses against alien cells placed in the body by surgical transplantation or arising in the body as incipient or established cancers. The practical problems that call for solution are to ensure that a kidney transplant is not rejected by the immune response or to accentuate an inadequate immune attack on a malignant tumour. Perhaps the clearest way to underline the human importance of both is to say that by 1970 about 3,500 kidney grafts had been successfully established for a year or longer essentially by using immunosuppressive drugs to damp down the immune response which in an untreated recipient would lead to rejection of the graft. But immunosuppression is a two-edged sword; it can also suppress immune responses against incipient cancer.

Amongst the 3,500 patients concerned there have been 36 cases of cancer arising *de novo*—only 2 or 3 would be expected—and 8 instances in which unsuspected cancer in the donor of the kidney had flourished in the kidney graft. In the absence of an immuno-suppressive drug, all experience says none of these accidental cancer transfers would have given rise to a tumour. Theory has, of course, gone along with practice and since Thomas threw out the first hint in 1959, there have been immunologists, including my-self, who feel that immunity, as we know it in mammals, could well have evolved to deal with cellular changes within the body rather than to improve the control of infectious disease.

One of the difficulties of modern immunology is the complexity it has developed and I find it correspondingly difficult to provide a simplified but reasonably accurate outline of the position for non-specialists interested in the biological side of medicine. My attempt will be greatly oversimplified—any professional immun-ologist could shoot it down with the greatest of ease—but it may be useful. It will be expressed in purely biological concepts of cells and tissues and chemical 'patterns' which are never defined in molecular terms.

Immunity can be defined for our purpose as the capacity to recognize the intrusion of material foreign to the body and to mobilize cells and cell products to help remove that particular sort of foreign material with greater speed and effectiveness. For this purpose, two systems of cells have been evolved. In the body they both arise as descendants of stem cells in the bone marrow.

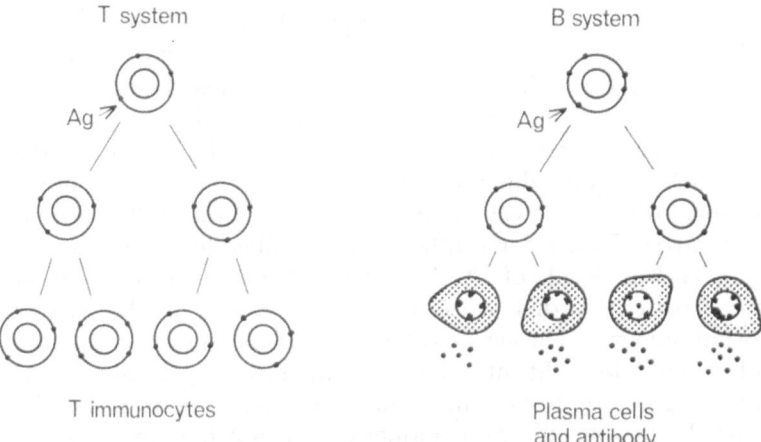

F IG. 7. The two systems of immune cells. The T system cells carry receptors (black dots) which are equivalent to antibody but they do not produce free antibody. The B system cells as they become plasma cells produce large amounts of antibody. Both types must be stimulated by antigen Ag if they are to multiply.

They have no immune properties until they have entered and multiplied in an appropriate organ. One such organ is the thymus (where calf sweetbreads come from!). There the cells develop and become adapted for their special role as immunocytes of the thymus-dependent or T series. The other site is known in the chicken but not in mammals: it may be somewhere along the intestinal tract from tonsil to appendix, it may be in the bone marrow itself. These cells become the B series of immunocytes.

Both B- and T-cells have patches of what it is convenient to call antibody on their surface and soon after an animal or a baby is born, both series have developed a great diversity of antibody patterns but only one pattern per cell. I shall deliberately say nothing of how those thousands of antibody patterns arise nor how any cells carrying patterns which might react with the body's own constituents are eliminated. The essence of the matter is that when a T-cell meets a chemical pattern X, usually on the surface of another cell, which it 'recognizes' because its own chemical pattern, its immune pattern, happens to fit the other in a lock and key, complementary pattern relationship, things start to happen. The T-cell is stimulated to proliferate and produce a family of descendant T-cells, a clone, all carrying the same immune pattern. When such cells now meet a group of cells carrying pattern X the T-cells attack and, if all goes well, eliminate their target cells. The B-cells have a different approach; their method of recognizing a foreign pattern in the body is probably basically similar but their response is quite different. They multiply and in the process change to a plasma cell clone. Basically a plasma cell is a highly specialized factory for synthesizing and liberating antibody protein, each molecule of which is identical and carries precisely the same pattern as that of the recognition groups on the ancestral B-immunocyte. The antibody has several functions the most useful of which is brought into play when the foreign pattern is carried by an invasive bacterium. When such an organism is lightly coated, 'opsonized', with antibody it is much more effectively taken in and destroyed by the phagocytic cells of blood and tissues.

The essential point to remember is that T-cells act *as* cells attaching themselves to and destroying their target cells. Their action is also spoken of as cell-mediated immunity and they are mostly concerned with foreign *cells*. The B-cells are primarily producers of soluble antibody and although antibody can be produced against almost any form of foreign pattern including those on transplanted or malignant cells, its main value is in protection against bacterial infections.

Perhaps the most illuminating example of modern principles of immunology in action is in relation to the prevention of 'Rh-disease' (haemolytic disease of the newborn). Probably everyone knows at least one couple who have been warned of the possibility that their child could be affected and the disease itself involves about one birth in every 400. It results essentially from destruction of the newborn infant's red blood cells by antibody which was produced by the mother during her pregnancy.

At first sight it seems completely unnatural that a normal pregnancy should give rise to a condition which may kill the child in its first weeks of life. To explain what happens we have to dig fairly deeply into the genetics of human blood groups. Most people at one time or another have been 'blood grouped' and know that their own group is O, A, B, or AB. They also appreciate how important it is to know this if they are to be involved in a blood transfusion either as blood donor or recipient patient. An O patient, for instance, has antibodies in his blood which will react

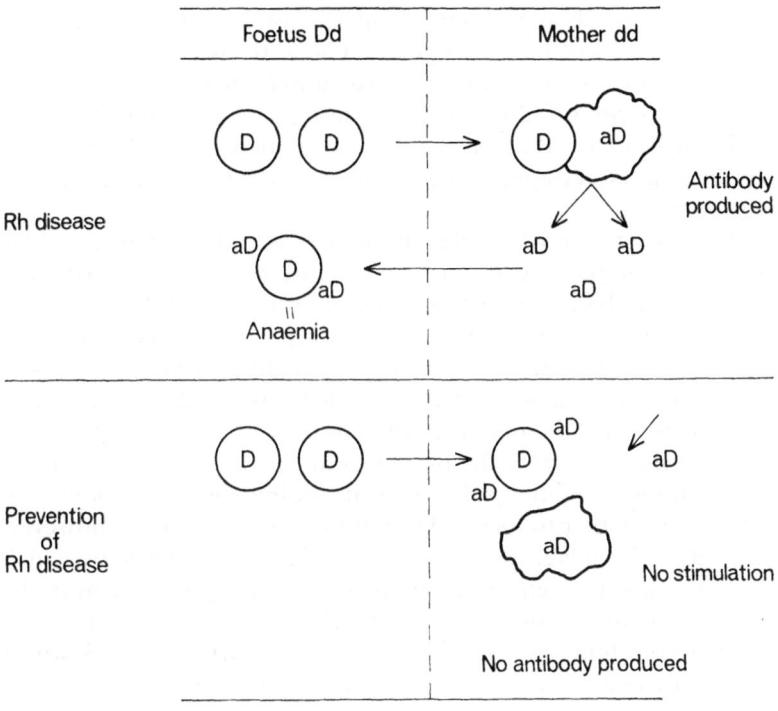

Foetus Dd	Mother dd

Rh disease

Antibody produced

Anaemia

Prevention
of
Rh disease

No stimulation

No antibody produced

To illustrate Rh disease

Circles: red cells   Irregular: immunocytes
D antigen (Rh+)   aD antibody against D

FIG. 8. The basis of Rh disease and its prevention.

with A or B red cells so that they are rapidly destroyed in the body. If he needs a transfusion it must be from a group O donor.

To say that a man's blood group is A means that on the surface of his red blood cells there are tiny patches of a chemical grouping (an antigen) which will react with an antibody, anti-A. There are many other sorts of antigen on red cells including a group spoken of as the Rh-system. For our purposes we can limit ourselves to one antigen D of the Rh-system, which determines whether an individual is 'Rh positive' or 'Rh negative'. This is a genetic difference and if we use the same letter D to represent the gene responsible for the presence of antigen D on the red cell and a little *d* to signify its absence, then persons *DD* or *Dd* will be Rh positive and those *dd* will be Rh negative. The antigen *D* differs from *A* and *B* in that no one normally has anti-*D* in his blood. Anti-*D* can only be produced if blood containing *D* from either *DD* or *Dd* individuals enters the circulation of someone who is *dd*. There the *D* antigen is recognized as foreign and antibody is produced against it.

It is easy to see where this discussion is leading. A man who is *DD* and Rh positive marries an Rh negative woman. All their children will be *Dd* and Rh positive and if the child's blood, before birth (or for the matter of that, at any time afterwards), enters the mother's circulation in sufficient amount she will produce anti-*D*. Until the very end of pregnancy the developing infant (the foetus) is well insulated immunologically speaking, from its mother. No blood cells pass across the barrier between the two blood circulations although soluble substances including some antibodies can pass from mother to foetus. During the process of birth, however, a sudden physiological metamorphosis has to take place by which the foetus, dependent on its mother's blood supply, becomes the infant responsible for its own continuing existence. The change is liable to result at one point in a brief but important breakdown of the insulation. At the time of birth when the uterus is contracting intermittently in the 'labour pains' minor haemorrhages are apt to occur at the junction of the two circulations (the placenta) and small amounts of the baby's blood leak into the mother's blood stream. Once this happens she is liable to become 'sensitized' against *D*. On the first occasion that this happens she is not likely to make any significant amount of anti-*D* but if antigen *D* again enters the circulation, she will.

So it happens that with each successive child—always *Dd* in a *dd* mother—she will be more and more likely to produce large amounts of anti-*D*. Often with the third child anti-*D* produced by the mother seeps into the foetus during the last month of pregnancy in sufficient amount to be dangerous. The antibody attaches itself to the *D* antigen on the baby's red cells and leads to their destruction. The baby is born acutely ill and anaemic with signs that blood destruction is still going on. In many cases the only way to save the baby's life is to wash the whole of the damaging antibody out of his circulation by exchange transfusion, i.e., by replacing his own blood with blood from compatible donors.

Within the last five years a method has been developed which is known to prevent sensitization of Rh negative mothers and which almost certainly can be applied to prevent more than 90 per cent of the cases of Rh-disease. At first hearing it sounds paradoxical to prevent the disease by an injection of the same anti-*D* which is responsible for the damage to the baby's red cells, yet this is the case. Any mother at risk, i.e., an Rh negative, *dd*, woman married to a *Dd* or *DD* husband is given a small injection of anti-*D* serum as soon as possible after the birth of each baby. The serum is at present obtained from women who have had babies with the disease but there are plans afoot to immunize *male* volunteers who are *dd* with *DD* blood and obtain serum from them when the antibody reaches a suitable level. There seems to be no reason why such artificially produced serum should not be just as effective.

There may be some subtle aspects of how the serum works which could only be discussed technically, but a simple explanation is available which is adequate for all practical purposes and may well be almost the whole story. When the serum is given soon after confinement the antibody rapidly latches on to the relatively small number of red cells from the baby that are in the mother's circulation. This allows these cells to be picked up at once by scavenging cells in the body. They are kept out of harm's way, as it were; few or none have an opportunity of meeting up with the special and rather rare cells in the mother which must initiate the process of sensitization and later antibody production. It is still too soon to say how effective the method will be—it only began to be used widely in 1968—but each successive report is good and most of those who are competent in haematology expect a rapid reduction in Rh-disease in all medically advanced countries over the next ten years.

There are volumes to be written about immunology—over the years I have written five myself!—but in this preliminary chapter there is only one additional point that I want to make. In that discussion of the Rh-disease, I spoke about *D* and *d* genes and the corresponding *D* and *d* antigens on red cells, also about anti-*D* cells and antibodies. I said nothing about what the molecular pattern of *D* was either as gene or as antigen or defined the antibody as anything but anti-*D* and in fact no one *can* define *D* or anti-*D* at the precise level of chemistry and physics. Yet with an unsophisticated experimentally based logic dealing with simple concepts like D and anti-D, we have been able to devise a life-saving procedure of the first importance.

Possibly it would be gratifying to know the precise structure of the reagents we work with in preventing disease but if more knowledge gives no more control over the human calamity which interests the ordinary man he will be tempted to ask, *Cui bono?* What's the good of it? In a real but perhaps faintly heretical sense this book is an attempt to answer that question and look at where medical science is moving in the last third of the twentieth century.

2

THE MARCH OF
MOLECULAR BIOLOGY

For three months in 1943–4 I was in America, interested primarily in research on infectious disease but eager to hear what was being done in all fields of microbiology. Many things impressed me but, in retrospect, two visits stand out. At the Rockefeller Institute in New York, Oswald Avery told me the story of how the transforming factor which could transfer an inheritable character from one strain of pneumococcus (a bacterium) to another was DNA (deoxyribonucleic acid). DNA was already well known to be a major component of cell nuclei and of bacterial viruses and was the favourite candidate for the chemical carrier of genetic information between cells and from one generation to the next. Avery's work was the first direct evidence that a definable substance could transfer inheritable information. No one thereafter doubted that DNA was the key to heredity.

The second visit was to Stanford to talk to Beadle and Tatum who at that time seemed to be doing most of their laboratory work in a basement corridor in the Medical School. They were studying the growth requirements and metabolism of a common mould, *Neurospora*. It was a mould with a simple form of bisexual reproduction and life-cycle that made it relatively simple to isolate the progeny of any hybridization. *Neurospora* is a versatile organism which can make almost every substance it needs from the small molecules of a simple nutrient solution. To make a moderately complex amino acid like tyrosine with ammonia and glucose as raw materials, requires a complex sequence of reactions within the cells of the mould by which substance A is changed by the action of enzyme x to substance B and then B to C by enzyme y and so on. One can symbolize the process as $- - - A \xrightarrow{x} B \xrightarrow{y} C \rightarrow - - -$ $\rightarrow K$ provided one remembers that at appropriate points other reaction chains come to interact with one we are considering.

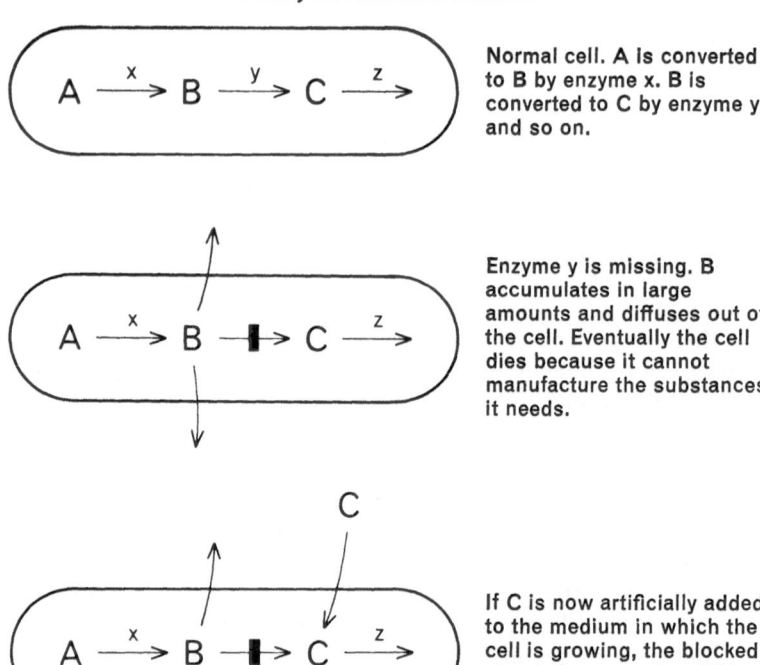

Normal cell. A is converted to B by enzyme x. B is converted to C by enzyme y and so on.

Enzyme y is missing. B accumulates in large amounts and diffuses out of the cell. Eventually the cell dies because it cannot manufacture the substances it needs.

If C is now artificially added to the medium in which the cell is growing, the blocked step is by-passed and the cell survives.

Fig. 9. The sequence of gene action.

Neurospora, like every other organism, is prone to mutations which may affect almost any of its qualities including its capacity to carry out these chemical sequences. If the end product of the ABC - - - K sequence is essential for growth, a mutation by which the step $A \xrightarrow{x} B$ is blocked will eventually mean the elimination of the mutant in the original environment. If, however, any one of the substances in the sequence B to K is added to the growth medium the mutant can now produce the vital substance K and will grow readily. Another characteristic of the mutant will be that since A is not being used up as fast as it is made, it will accumulate in exceptionally large amount in the culture where it can be measured by appropriate chemical tests. These two sets of characteristics made it a relatively straightforward matter to define the various synthetic sequences.

Pushing the matter further, Beadle and Tatum showed that the enzyme that was responsible for the blocked step *A* to *B* was actually absent or functionally inert in the mutant. Gradually this sort of work led them to the famous generalization 'one gene, one enzyme'. They postulated that a gene, as defined genetically by hybridization experiments, was directly responsible for the functional quality of one particular enzyme as defined biochemically. Two major sciences had found common meeting ground. Having regard to the fact that all enzymes are proteins, this pointed very directly to the likelihood of a direct relationship between the gene and protein synthesis.

Both Avery's work on the pneumococcus DNA and Beadle's and Tatum's on *Neurospora* were preceded by and led up to by years of research in many laboratories. Nevertheless, I believe that quite apart from the fact that I made personal contact with the scientists concerned in 1943, these are two of the classic milestones in the development of molecular biology. In both sets of experiments, genetics was directly implicated in biochemistry and in both, micro-organisms were being used. Since then, molecular biology and biochemical genetics have become synonymous and all the great generalizations of molecular biology have been worked out on micro-organisms, usually bacteria, but moulds, like *Neurospora*, and the bacterial viruses (bacteriophages) have both played a major part as well.

I believe that I can claim to have been aware as early as any other microbiologist, of the potentialities of genetic work with bacteria and viruses. In 1930 I wrote that 'the changes (i.e., the development of bacterial resistance to phages) seem to be much more comparable to losses and reassortments of Mendelian genes than to the development of active immunity in mammals'. To the best of my knowledge the statement made in the Dunham Lectures of 1944: 'That heritable variations in bacteria and viruses arise by a process of discontinuous mutation essentially similar to gene mutation in higher forms and that the mass transformation of a strain as observed in practice is the result of selective survival and overgrowth of one or more mutant types' (Burnet, 1945, p. 14) had not previously been made.

It gives a vivid realization of how young a science is molecular biology to find on the next page 'One would hazard the prophecy (in January 1944) that when "academic" research is again permissible the study of micro-organismal genetics *will* show that bacterial hereditary mechanisms are accurately quantized and in addition provide data of fundamental impoitance for the interpretation of organic evolution.'

There was never a prediction that was so abundantly and rapidly fulfilled.

In this book I am concerned with genetic ideas as they impinge on human affairs and primarily with how genetic changes in man himself can be associated with disability or disease. But, as I have already said, most of the really fundamental concepts of genetics have been worked out with micro-organisms and if one is to obtain a relatively clear, if rather superficial, understanding of human genetics it will be necessary to look rather carefully at the special virtues of bacteria and other micro-organisms for such work.

Before doing so, however, it is right to pay brief tribute to a physician who in 1909 grasped the essentials of the one gene, one enzyme, dogma from studying what he called inborn errors of metabolism in man. Sir Archibald Garrod, a London physician specially interested in paediatrics, wrote on albinism, alcaptonuria, cystinuria, and pentosuria, all conditions in which a major genetic abnormality of metabolism was consistent with prolonged survival of the individual. As Garrod predicted, very many more examples of such metabolic anomalies have been observed since, and several of them will be discussed in Chapter 6. Here I will just quote two sentences from Garrod (second edition, 1923): '. . . each successive step in the building up and breaking down not merely of proteins, carbohydrates and fats in general, but even of individual fractions . . . is the work of special enzymes set apart for each particular purpose' and '. . . the most probable cause (of the inborn errors) is the congenital lack of some particular enzyme in the absence of which a step is missed and some normal metabolic change fails to be brought about'.

The resemblance to Beadle's and Tatum's approach is obvious but it is easier to work with bacteria and we can return to bacterial genetics for a few pages.

For obvious reasons my account of the development of bacterial genetics and how it led to modern molecular biology will have to be a superficial one. Within its limits, the most important of which is the attempt to describe the essentials without making use of organic chemistry, I believe it comes close to accepted teaching. For readers with a moderate grounding in biochemistry a much more satisfactory account will be found in J. D. Watson's *Molecular Biology of the Gene*, published in 1965.

BACTERIAL GENETICS

Let us take the most commonly used micro-organism as an example, the bacterium *Escherichia coli*. In working with bacteria we use the same word as the livestock breeder, a strain, to label a culture with genetic characteristics that interest us. In genetic work with bacteria, two strains of *E. coli* have been specially studied both primarily because of their behaviour in relation to bacterial viruses. There are vast numbers of bacterial viruses, also called bacteriophages or phages, in all situations where bacteria are active in nature. They are in as wide a variety as the viruses which attack plants and animals and critical study of some selected strains has brought some of the most exciting discoveries in molecular biology.

E. coli B was the organism used as host for what became a standard group of bacterial viruses, and *E. coli K12* became of special interest because it was lysogenic, i.e., carried a virus λ (lambda) which under special circumstances could be activated but was normally undetectable. Both *B* and *K12* were 'old laboratory cultures' isolated many years before, either from human faeces or from one of the abscesses or inflammatory areas that bacteria of this type may cause. For work on bacterial viruses or on bacterial metabolism it was quite immaterial whether the bacterial strain had any of the characters which would allow it to prosper in the human intestine or provoke an appendical abscess. All that was necessary was that it should proliferate readily in a simple chemical medium, present no danger to laboratory workers and be highly susceptible to the standard bacteriophages. Once the two *coli* strains had been chosen and found suitable, there was every reason for retaining them as standard strains indefinitely. It is immaterial that there were probably dozens of other species of bacteria and thousands of individual strains which could have served just as well.

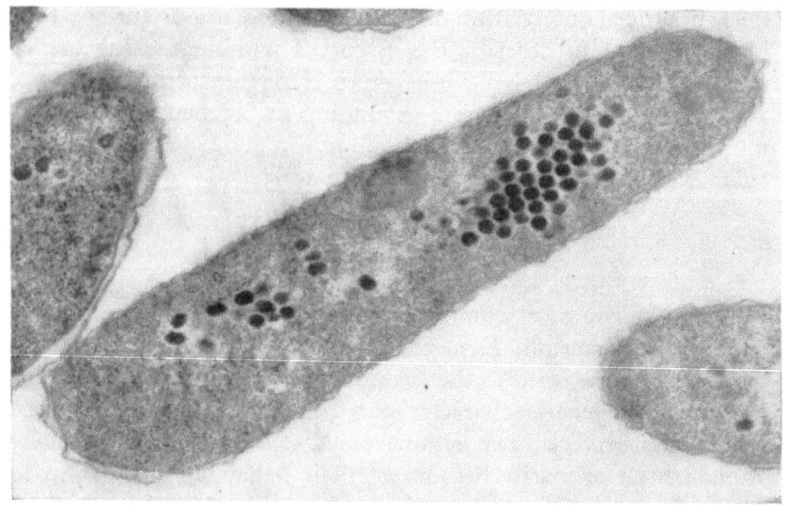

FIG. 10. Electron-micrograph showing bacterial viruses in the host
bacterium (×34,000 approx) (Kellenberger, Geneva).

Escherichia coli is a typical rod-shaped bacterium roughly 3 μm
long by 1 μm in diameter (1 μm being $\frac{1}{1000}$ of a millimetre). It
contains in each individual rod, all the standard components of
living substance, protein, fat and carbohydrate, enzymes, vitamins, DNA, and RNA. It can grow in the presence of oxygen or
without it, necessarily switching aspects of its metabolism when
it changes from one state to the other. Every one of its components can be synthesized from a solution containing glucose
as a source of energy, an ammonium salt to provide nitrogen and
a salt mixture to provide the other necessary elements. It is of
special interest that all the twenty standard amino acids of
protein and the five purine and pyrimidine bases of nucleic
acid can be built up from these simplest of all possible nutrients.
To carry out this fantastic feat of chemistry, some hundreds of
enzymes must be provided in appropriate concentration and
spatial distribution.

This chemical versatility of *E. coli* is particularly convenient
for biochemical-genetic work of the general type that Beadle
and Tatum were doing with *Neurospora*. In the process which
through the $A \rightarrow B \rightarrow C$ series runs from glucose and ammonia

to an amino acid like tyrosine, there may be a dozen steps but each successive product remains something with a small molecule which can easily diffuse into the bacterium if it is added to the medium. Similarly, if too much is present inside, it can diffuse out. Just as in *Neurospora*, if the $\rightarrow B \xrightarrow{x} C \rightarrow$ stage in some vitally important synthesis is blocked by a mutation that inactivates enzyme x, then the bacterium will not grow unless ready-made C is added to the medium and the newly synthesized B, which cannot be used, will escape out into the medium in abnormal excess.

The next important advantage of bacteria is the possibility of obtaining unlimited amounts of genetically uniform material. With well established techniques it is possible to obtain kilograms of dried bacteria in which 99·9 per cent at least, are of uniform genetic character. The rest will have undergone some mutation during the process of growing the culture. A kilogram of dried bacteria contains something of the order or 10^{15} (i.e., a million American billions) individuals. This means that even if there are only ten molecules or some type we are interested in, per bacterium—a particular enzyme for example—enough could be extracted for effective microchemical characterization. It must never be forgotten that *all* chemical work must be done with a large population of uniform molecules in an environment effectively free from other types of molecule which could be confused with the one under study. Perhaps the most important application of this principle is in relation to information-carrying nucleic acids. The DNA of a bacterium has the responsibility of carrying the 'blueprints' needed for the construction of some hundreds of proteins and, in 1971, is too complex for sequence studies and synthesis. Nevertheless it can easily be obtained in pure form and in sufficient amount to allow a wide variety of useful investigations of its activities.

Still further advantages of the same general character can be obtained by the use of a bacterial virus. The bacteriophages can be considered in the first instance as extremely minute organisms parasitic on bacteria. The commonly studied types, the DNA bacteriophages, are still highly complex structures but there are smaller and simpler RNA bacteriophages which in the last few years have become of special interest to molecular biologists since they seem to have reduced the essentials of life to the absolute limit. Each unit has a single thread of RNA with genes or 'blueprints' for just three proteins, two of which form part of the phage particle structure while the third is an enzyme needed to allow doubling of the RNA.

It is basically correct to picture the activity of either DNA or RNA phage as a sequence in which the phage particle attaches to the bacterial surface and inserts its nucleic acid into the bacterial substance. There the nucleic acid seizes on the protein-synthesizing machinery of the host bacterium, the ribosomes and the pool of amino acids and transfer-RNA, and forces it to produce phage proteins, including enzymes which make it possible for the phage nucleic acid to duplicate itself, also at the expense of the necessary chemical building blocks that the bacterium has made for its own use. New phage particles construct themselves as the needed material accumulates, while all normal growth activities of the bacterium stop and disintegration begins. Finally, the 'skin' of the bacterium breaks and a brood of a hundred or more new phage particles is liberated to continue the process wherever a susceptible bacterium can be found.

From 1945 onwards the approach toward understanding the functions of the nucleic acids in relation to protein synthesis was rapid. Only the important steps will be mentioned and the reader interested predominantly in medical and social implications is advised to skim lightly over the rest of this chapter. The understanding of the process of protein synthesis in the cell has advanced enormously in the last decade but it is still a highly complex story.

It is obvious that before one can discuss protein synthesis the standard chemical structure of proteins and of nucleic acids must be known. Proteins have been known for many years to be constructed in the form of peptide chains, linear sequences in which amino acids are linked by —CO—NH— groupings to form polypeptide chains. With only minor exceptions all proteins are made up from twenty different amino acids and it is convenient and logical to regard these 20 as an alphabet from which can be built up 'words and sentences' which have a meaning for the function of the protein. A portion of a protein could be expressed, for example, as

. . . —B—P—R—E—B—K—L—O—F— . . .

Most proteins have approximately 200–1,000 amino acids per molecule.

Nucleic acids are more complex but again they are linear sequences, this time of nucleotides. Again, there is no need to particularize the nature of nucleotides. From our point of view they can be simply given names from a five-letter alphabet A.C.G.T.U. Nucleotide chains are single or double-stranded. A single strand could be represented:

—A—C—C—G—T—T—A—G—C—T—

in DNA or

—A—C—C—G—U—U—A—G—C—U—

in RNA where U is equivalent to T in DNA.

For double-stranded DNA, the double helix of Watson and Crick, there are certain simple rules that everyone knows and without showing the helical character, a portion of double-strand could be represented:

—A—C—C—G—T—T—A—G—C—T—
—T—G—G—C—A—A—T—C—G—A—

The rule is that A and T always pair as do G and C.

The next step was to elucidate the broad relationships between nucleic acids DNA and RNA and protein synthesis. Without spending any time on the history of discovery there is now available a simple scheme which can be stated and shown diagramatically.

1. Double-stranded DNA is the primary carrier of genetic information. It multiplies by unwinding and building on to each single strand the complementary sequence of nucleotides.

2. For protein synthesis an unwound strand of DNA attracts to itself nucleotides of the A.C.G.U. series to produce a single-strand RNA sequence that, as it were, transcribes the DNA information. It is called messenger-RNA or m-RNA.

3. Messenger-RNA becomes attached to ribosomes, minute granules made up of protein and another type of RNA, which function to direct the 'translation' of the m-RNA sequence into an amino acid sequence in a way that could be remotely compared with the way a tape recorder translates sound into a sequence of magnetic configurations in the tape or vice versa.

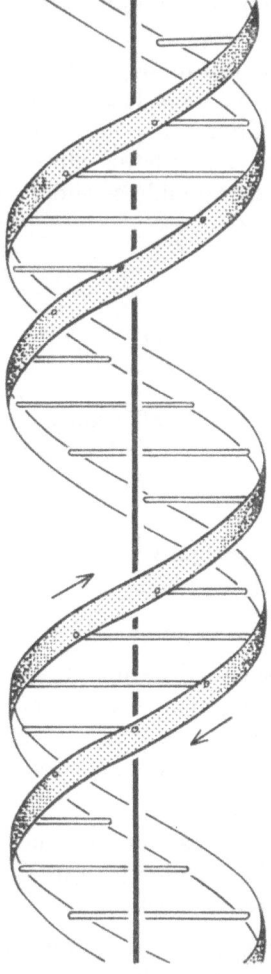

FIG. 11. The double helix of Watson and Crick. This figure is purely diagrammatic. The two ribbons symbolize the two phosphate chains, and the horizontal rods the pairs of bases holding the chains together. The vertical line marks the fibre axis (*Nature*, 1953).

4. Protein synthesis from the surrounding pool of amino acids is carried out by a collection of small RNA molecules, called transfer-RNAs, twenty of them, one for each type of amino acid. Each transfer-RNA molecule can be said with approximate truth to be able to recognize with one end a particular triad of nucleotides, AUC for instance, and with the other end the corresponding amino acid, B perhaps (i.e., if B represents isoleucine). In crude terms the transfer-RNA attaches for a

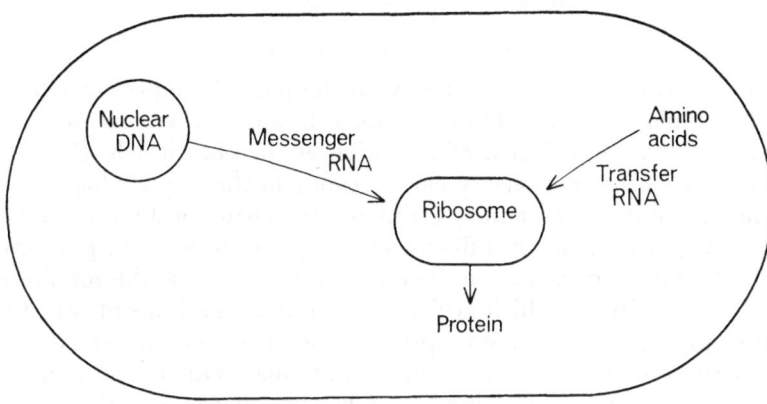

FIG. 12. An outline of protein synthesis.

moment to the nucleotide triad of m-RNA as it moves over the ribosome reading head, and at that moment transfers the amino acid on its other end to the growing peptide chain that will become the protein proper to the gene concerned. This provides a means by which the m-RNA is 'read' from one end to the other with the concomitant construction of the right protein chain.

All the essential aspects of these processes can be carried out in the test-tube provided the building blocks, enzymes and ribosomes, are provided as well as the nucleic acid to give the primary informational sequence.

It is obvious from this account of the process that there is a crucial need for knowing 'the genetic code', i.e., the rules for translating a nucleotide sequence into a protein sequence. In addition to making a table which says AUC—isoleucine and so on, there are various other rules about 'syntax and punctuation'; where to start and where to end the protein chain, for instance. The genetic code is now available in tables as precise as the multiplication table and—a very important point—it is known to be the same code for every organism from RNA virus to man. If ever some lowly organism is brought back from Mars the basic question that it will be asked by the biochemists is whether it is constructed under the same genetic code as terrestrial organisms.

EVOLUTION OF PROTEINS

We are going to be concerned with the possible impact of molecular biology on the evolution of man. It is vital, therefore, to look at what has been learnt of evolution at the chemical level. The approach has a reasonably close analogy to the way zoologists in the late nineteenth century compared the anatomical structure of homologous organs in different living species to gain insight into the evolutionary sequence. The classical example is the forelimb of the vertebrates which evolved from the pectoral fins of fish. In the amphibians it took on a primitive standard pattern which has persisted in very much the same form to man. Other evolutionary paths, however, led towards highly specialized equivalents, in birds, bats, horses, and seals, for instance, or its complete loss in the snakes and slow worms. Wherever there is a forelimb, however, it is possible to recognize its homology with the primitive pattern.

At the biochemical level one trades on the broad uniformity of metabolic processes in living organisms. Haemoglobin, the red pigment of the blood is present in all vertebrates, with one or two peculiar exceptions, and in many invertebrates. All organisms have cytochrome c and there are many other enzymes which are homologous through a very wide range of living forms. Most of the detailed study has made use of haemoglobin or cytochrome c but what has been recognized in them appears to hold also for any other proteins studied. Haemoglobin is a four-chained protein, which introduces unnecessary complication to the discussion, and it is probably simplest to start with an unspecified protein behaving in evolution as cytochrome c or a single haemoglobin chain. If we take such a series as man, monkey, mouse, fish, insect, yeast, alga, flowering plant, and examine our homologous protein by determining the number and sequence of amino acids in the protein chain, the results take the following form:

There is a certain recognizable similarity throughout. We might find, for instance, that all have between 120 and 140 amino acids and with a little ingenuity to allow for missing units or groups it can be seen that there are numerous sequences in common:

BD	EF	MELONP	BRO	SYLEMONH	P	SF	- - - 24
BD	YX	MELONP	R - -	SYLEMONH	E	SF	- - - 22

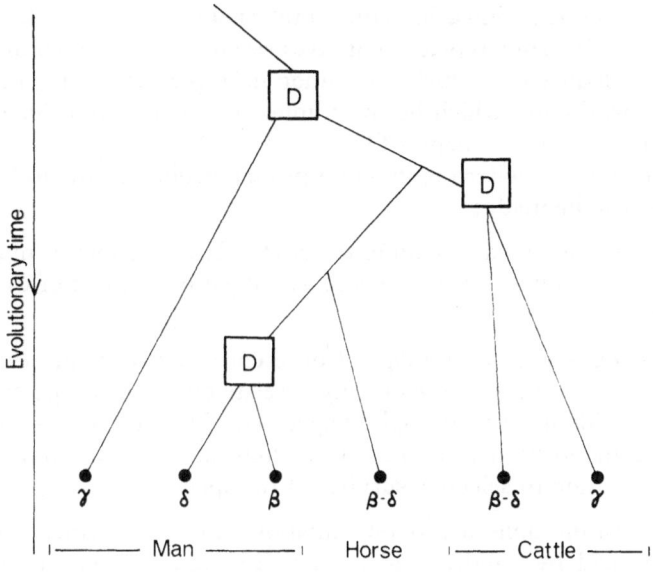

Contemporary haemoglobins

FIG. 13. A diagram from Zuckermann and Pauling show how gene duplications probably occurred in the evolution of haemoglobin. (E. Zuckermann and J. L. Pauling, *Evolving Genes and Proteins,* ed. Bryson J. Vogel (New York: Academic Press, 1965), 156.)

The two sequences shown of 24 and 22 amino acids are clearly homologous since 18 of them correspond, and both start at the left-hand end, with BD.

The next point is that the differences are roughly proportional to the evolutionary distance between the forms concerned. There are few differences between man and monkey, even less between man and chimpanzee but it may be quite difficult to find more than a few sequences in common between man and beast.

The next finding of evolutionary significance is that for any species in a freely interbreeding population the vast majority of individuals give proteins that conform completely to the standard form. Man is almost the only mammal who has been examined extensively on this point mainly in regard to haemoglobins. A small proportion of human beings, however, have been found to have haemoglobin which is chemically abnormal usually in the sense that one amino acid in one of the chains has been replaced by another. One such replacement gives rise to a well-defined disease, sickle cell anaemia, which is common in tropical (malarial) regions of the world and which has been much discussed from the evolutionary angle (see Chapter 6).

To sum up modern opinion on protein evolution, the following points can be made:

1. Every functional protein found as standard in a species must be adequately suited for its purpose as judged by the test of over-all survival.

2. The extremely wide range of differences between species indicates that for most proteins only a relatively small proportion of amino acids need to be rigidly specified. The distribution of the rest seems to be determined by random factors which have little or no relation to selective survival of the species.

3. Most mutations are point mutations, i.e., replacement of one amino acid by another and most point mutations can be interpreted as depending on a single change in the nucleotide triad (the codon) which decides the amino acid. For instance, if AUC becomes AUG, isoleucine is replaced by methionine.

4. It is possible, though far from established for any higher form, that the first step in the expression of *all* inheritable characters is the synthesis of proteins with the necessary consequence that all mutations act primarily by disturbing the sequence of some protein.

GENE DUPLICATION

There is much more, however, to be learnt from the pattern of amino acid sequence in proteins. For instance in speaking of haemoglobin evolution, I merely mentioned in passing that it was a protein made up of four polypeptide chains.

If we go into a little more detail, one or two points of general significance can be made. In the haemoglobin molecule the four chains comprise two of α pattern, two of a different β pattern and for each type there is a separate gene. Despite this the α and β chains have many corresponding sequences of amino acids and must have somehow arisen from a common ancestral pattern. To make the matter even more complex there is a human haemoglobin present before birth and called foetal haemoglobin in which there is another different but related chain γ replacing the two βs another found only very early in embryonic life (ε) and a small proportion of yet another present in adult life (δ). Finally there is a functionally different protein in muscle, myoglobin which is another single chain polypeptide, again clearly related to α and β chains.

This introduces the important concept of gene duplication. The differences between the haemoglobins of different species and at different stages of development in the same species make sense only if all the unit chains are in a real sense descendants of a single pattern specified by a single primordial gene. That gene carried the information for a polypeptide chain of about 140 units. It was always prone to point-mutation by which one 'letter' is replaced by another and every few million years a new pattern resulting from such a modification was taken over by evolution as the standard form. Much more rarely the gene duplicated and descendants with two genes were in some way fitter than those with one. From now on, the two genes were autonomous each subject to point-mutation and more rarely to further duplication. So it comes about that in all normal human beings there are at least six genes for a group or protein chains (myoglobin, $\alpha, \beta, \gamma, \delta$, and ε) descended from the primordial gene. In the course of evolution elaborate arrangements—'switchgear' is one name for them—have come into being to ensure that each gene comes into action at the right time and in the right cells and that the appropriate mechanism to make the composite molecules $\alpha_2 \beta_2$ and so on, can function.

It is now becoming clear that processes of this sort must have played a basic role in the evolution of more and more complex organisms and that they are still going on. When any body protein is really studied in depth it is rare not to find that there are several molecular forms with related but not identical functions plus some rare anomalous types which may or may not be associated with a related disease.

As an immunologist the protein I am most interested in is antibody, or immunoglobulin. We use the first word if we are interested in the biological function of the protein, the second if we are thinking about its chemical structure. Otherwise, antibody and immunoglobulin are synonymous.

The chemistry of antibodies has become extremely complicated and I shall only refer very briefly to the structure of the commonest type of immunoglobulin which is called IgG. Like haemoglobin it is built of four polypeptide chains, two heavy (H) and two light (L). It is a two-ended molecule and at each end there is co-operation by parts of L and H chains to form the combining site by which an antibody 'recognizes' and unites with the corresponding antigen.

Current theory suggests that the processes by which a single individual can produce such an extraordinarily wide diversity of distinct antibodies—perhaps 10,000 or more—are much the same as have been concerned with the long-term evolution of proteins. It is what might be called a hotted-up version so that changes more or less equivalent to ones normally requiring millions of years of evolution can take place in the period between conception and adolescence. It is too complex a story to elaborate. All that is relevant here is that the immune system is probably the most extensive and important example of gene duplication in vertebrates.

THE FUTURE OF MOLECULAR BIOLOGY

For one who is not an active molecular biologist and must obtain his information from secondary sources, these dozen pages seem to cover most of what is known at present which is conceivably relevant to any medical, industrial, or military applications of molecular biology. It is desirable, however, to look at present possibilities of advance.

In 1971 the principles for chemical sequencing of nucleotides in any segment of functionally identifiable DNA or RNA are known and the sequence for several transfer-RNAs which contain approximately eighty nucleotides have been reported. Quite recently the DNA gene that is responsible for one of the transfer-RNAs has actually been synthesized—but it is a very small gene. Segments of bacteriophage m-RNA have been shown to correspond in translation to substantial sequences of coat protein as isolated from the phage, so providing the most direct possible proof of the accuracy of the genetic code. As things stand at present, one gets the impression that those at the growing edge of molecular biology are looking not so much for what will bear on practical matters but for some spectacular sounding advance that might attract what one reviewer of *The Double Helix* called the persimmon—a Nobel prize.

The next achievement likely to follow the sequence of prizes in molecular biology that started with Watson, Crick, and Wilkins, is the complete specification of an RNA bacteriophage in chemical terms. There is still some distance to go and there may be some considerable technical hurdles still to be cleared. The sequence and three-dimensional structure of the three proteins can in principle be determined if sufficient purified material can be provided but it is well to remember how many years it took for simpler proteins like insulin and myoglobin to be fully characterized. Nucleotide sequences of the three units of RNA—cistrons they are called—which specify the three proteins could be sequenced in principle from the structure of the proteins and with this guide the chemical analysis should not be difficult. There is still, however, 20 or 30 per cent of the RNA which seems to have operational rather than 'blueprint' responsibilities. Its exact function is in doubt but almost certainly it is in part at least, concerned with recognizing the host components which it must subvert to its own uses. Such understanding, however, is not necessary for the complete specification of structure.

Living substance, even the simplest, is the accumulated wisdom of more than 3,000 million years of evolution on earth and its subtleties will probably always remain beyond the understanding of another product of evolution like ourselves. To know the structure of an RNA virus may win a group of people a Nobel prize but it will still be far from an understanding of what happens when the phage enters, multiplies in, and dissolves the bacterium. And that is the simplest of all interactions between two species of organism. I once wrote a book with the title *Virus as Organism* and many people thought it a good book and a good title. But no professional virologist, nowadays necessarily steeped in molecular biology, will allow me to call a virus an organism. They are perfectly right if, like Humpty Dumpty, they say of organism that 'it means just what we choose it to mean—neither more nor less'. The relevant definition in the *Oxford English Dictionary* is: 'An organized body consisting of mutually connected and dependent parts constituted to share a common life.' This may seem to fit an RNA virus just as well as *E. coli* or an elephant but following André Lwoff, the virologists demand that an organism must not be wholly dependent on some other organism for its existence. An RNA virus can from one point of view be regarded as no more than a set of instructions to cause the machine that is a complete organism to destroy itself. This is the modern approach, and it indicates the next direction where distinction in biochemical scholarship may be won.

I have mentioned the necessity for part of the virus RNA to 'recognize' the metabolic machines the ribosomes of the host. Recognition has become almost a technical word in biochemistry and particularly when we are dealing with immunology. An antigen recognizes the one specific antibody which will react with it. In similar fashion a given bacteriophage can only multiply in and dissolve a limited range of bacterial species. It must recognize the right host at two levels. It must find the right vantage point on the bacterial surface which will allow it to enter and once the RNA has been freed from its coat it must recognize that the host ribosomes are suitable for making all three proteins. Once we know the sequential structure of the so-called initiation groups on phage RNA when it functions as messenger-RNA it should be possible to approach the detailed structure of the ribosome.

I have already compared the ribosome to the recording head of a tape-recorder by which information coming to it on the long threads of messenger-RNA from the organism or cell's central library is translated into the amino acid chains of protein. It is not far from the reality to picture the intruding tape of the virus as having the appropriate shape and twist that will allow it easily to be threaded on. Once it recognizes the recording head as appropriate it moves in and takes over the establishment. This may be enough to make it clear why I believe that the second great advance on the horizon of molecular biology is an adequate description of the ribosome and the precise mechanism of translation from messenger-RNA to protein. For a variety of technical reasons it will probably prove easier to analyse the process when the alien virus 'tape' is using the ribosomes than when they are fulfilling their normal function of translating legitimate messages.

Rightly or wrongly I think that with those two discoveries, Nobel prizes in molecular biology will stop. The scientists in that field will have an infinite number of things that they could do. There are countless other species of micro-organism to be studied in the same ways that *E. coli B* and its phages have been. Many of them may have diverged in their evolution from *E. coli*'s ancestors a thousand million years ago and equally detailed study would no doubt give a similar general pattern but for every new type tested there would be deviations from pattern to be recognized, puzzled out, and eventually understood. With *E. coli* itself almost any sequence of metabolic processes or any single enzyme could be made the theme for a near lifetime of good scientific work. But this would not bring a molecular understanding of *E. coli* much nearer. If it took x years to gain a good understanding of one system or one enzyme, the time required to deal fully with all the enzymes (perhaps two hundred) and their interactions in *E. coli* would take at least x centuries if it could be done at all. My favourite phrase for the situation is that we are up against an asymptotic brick wall. Progress in understanding can continue for ever but the cost/benefit ratio becomes less and less attractive.

Things may change for reasons I shall discuss in a later chapter but, given the current traditions and motivations of modern biological laboratories, I do not think that first-rate workers will be drawn to work indefinitely trying to push back those frustrating walls. If understanding and the prestige it brings are not forthcoming they will move elsewhere.

3

CELLULAR MANIPULATIONS

One way of dividing the subject matter of biology into segments that are convenient for academic handling is to say that it can be approached at three levels, (1) the molecular level, (2) the cellular level, and (3) at the level of the organism as a whole. There are various intermediate positions and more interrelationships but generally the division is a good one. Having outlined the position of molecular biology we must now provide a similar, rather superficial picture of what is going on in the realm of cytology and cell genetics. For our present purpose this is important, as the layman with a minor interest in biology and its impact on human affairs is very liable to find himself confused about the boundaries between the realms of the biochemist on the one hand and the cytologist on the other.

In this chapter I am primarily concerned with *human* cells, though it will often be necessary to refer to experimental work in laboratory animals if the human applications are to be made clear. Cytology is concerned with the behaviour of cells as units. This includes the germ cells which is a term used to cover not only the actual egg and sperm cells but also the ancestral cell lines which were segregated for their reproductive role early in embryonic life. For the most part, however, somatic cells will be at the centre of interest. 'Somatic' in this sense is a word whose only real function is a negative one, used to make it plain that the cells we are talking about are not germ cells. They include every other type of cell to be found in the body, specialized like muscle or nerve cells or relatively unspecialized like the white cells of the blood. Every organism, man included, is made up of cells and cell products of which the solid substance of bone, the fibres that give strength and elasticity to tissues, and the fluids of the body, are the most important. All cells, the germ cells as well as all the rest, arise by the growth and division of a parental cell into two daughter cells. The fertilized ovum divides into two and for a short time there is a simple multiplication by binary fission, 2, 4, 8, etc., until a ball of 32 or 64 cells is produced. From then on there enter all the complications of differentiation and development but there is never a break in the continuity of the process of cell division.

Discussion of possible human implications of modern cytology can be divided naturally into possibilities that concern the sex cells and those involving somatic cells. It is a common and, I believe, correct statement to say that all somatic cells of the body contain all the 'information' that is present in the fertilized ovum, the zygote. I have already found myself using the word 'information' in its biological sense on earlier pages but it seems appropriate to look at it a little more critically at this stage. Information has a distinctly different slant when we use it in a biological context. It is technically possible to implant a fertilized ovum of a mouse of strain *A* in the uterus of a strain *B* mouse, the zygote will develop and a mouse of *A* type with no sign of *B* characteristics will develop. It is legitimate, therefore, to say that at least all the information that differentiates mouse strains *A*, *B*, *C*, etc., is present in the fertilized ovum. Later on in this chapter I shall refer to experiments with frogs which establish that the *whole* of the information that allows an adult frog to develop is in the *nucleus* of the zygote or of any of its immediate descendants.

There is a real analogy to the building of a factory in regard to the use of biological information. I have already casually equated DNA with blueprints but a comparison with the construction of a factory will show that there is much more to DNA than that. There are plans and specifications—information on paper—for the factory buildings, and there is a more complex documentation for the machinery to be installed, flow-sheets for fuel, raw material, subcontractors' parts and so on, estimates for personnel and plans to obtain and train them and, finally, financial budgets and estimates of ultimate profitability. All this can be put on paper and when the factory is built and running it may seem that everything about it had been clearly laid out in the documents. One important thing that is *not* there, however, is the knowledge and experience of the men who translated the blueprints, etc., into the functioning organism of the factory. In most writings on genetics and molecular biology we are interested in the specification in the gene for the protein that is produced and which we can analyse. There is infinitely less understood about the 'managerial' aspects of when and how much of protein X is produced and how its production is correlated with the changing needs of the developing organism. Even more difficult is it to understand how all the information can, as it were, be distributed to male and female sex cells in such a fashion that a working whole will be reconstituted by appropriate fusion with an opposite number. Nothing remotely analogous is to be seen in factory building or any other non-biological model.

In many ways the sex cells provide the only approach we have to understanding and attempting to modify genetic processes. Male (sperm) and female (ova) sex cells are almost equivalent in their content of information in the sense that we have been using that term, but for fairly obvious reasons the sperm is much more accessible for detailed study than the ovum, and discussion will be almost limited to the spermatozoa.

THE SPERM CELLS

As cells, spermatozoa are in a class by themselves. To take a human sperm as a typical enough example we have a cell with practically no cytoplasm and a small nucleus of solidly packed chromosomes which makes up the whole of the head of the spermatozoon. The rest of the cell is a tail that sends it swimming along at a millimetre or two per minute and a mid-piece which joins head to tail and in a sense provides the motor power for the tail. It is an actively mobile cell, in many ways resembling a free living micro-organism, whose only function is to race in the direction where an ovum may be waiting to be fertilized—and to be the first of some 300 million competitors to reach that ovum. The head of the human spermatozoon is the most concentrated accumulation of information in the universe. In that infinitesimal speck of organized nucleic acid and protein there is the information to create half a man. In all probability there is so much mutual redundancy of information in ovum and sperm that either could probably provide the specification for 90 per cent of the organism that arises from their fusion.

There is a curious contrast between the male and the female sex cells in any mammal including man. Spermatozoa are extremely small and are produced in fantastically large numbers, 300 million in a single ejaculation. The ova are laid down before birth to provide the few hundred needed for one to mature and be liberated each month from the menarche to the menopause. When mature it is a large cell, visible with a hand lens, which contains a large supply of nucleic acid building blocks and other nutrients to allow of all the activities which will follow fertilization.

Scientists, like the rest of humanity, are interested in sex and in the last ten years the biochemists have been responsible for one of the greatest biological and moral revolutions in the history of our species. The full implications of the contraceptive pill are yet to be seen but it is here and it is effective. It may be replaced by something better or more convenient but the revolutionary implication will remain that sexual activity is now readily dissociable from reproduction. Reproduction is now something to be undertaken when desired, soon it may be something not to be undertaken without permission from authority.

In this book I am not concerned with contraception which is from the scientific and technological angle a fully accomplished fact. What I am concerned with is the possibility of further extensions of control in the field of reproduction. The first is the possibility of application to human beings of the principles of artificial insemination which have revolutionized cattle breeding. The second is in regard to the possibility of ensuring that the next baby is of the desired sex. Both possibilities would have been inconceivable in the days before the dissociation of sex from reproduction. With the acceptance of the fact that the deeply based gratification of a satisfactory sex life can be separated entirely from a woman's reproductive experience, the way is open for deliberate medico-scientific intervention as a means of initiating pregnancy. There may be no real justification for it, or no adequate technical expertise but it is no longer unthinkable.

Here the only legitimate approach is to discuss wholly at the biological level the possibilities and the difficulties in the way of their achievement.

ARTIFICIAL INSEMINATION

Artificial insemination has become virtually standard practice in dairy cattle breeding in the last twenty to thirty years. An elaborate technology has been developed and a bull with the natural capacity to serve 30 to 50 cows annually can now father more than 2,000 calves—I have seen 10,000 mentioned in one publication! Semen appropriately diluted in saline solution containing glycerol and frozen to the temperature of dry ice — 70 °C can keep bull spermatozoa in viable form almost indefinitely, certainly for four years. This has allowed transport of bull semen by air to any part of the globe.

The modern objective in breeding dairy cattle is to increase the total yield of milk and butter fat for each lactation period; other requirements are all secondary to this. Progeny testing is now made the main criterion of a bull's worth. If he can regularly produce daughters with a better record of production than their dams, his services will be in strong demand. Such proof takes several years which is a substantial part of a bull's period of sexual vigour and it would be of obvious value for much of his early output of semen to be maintained in the frozen but viable condition until early progeny tests had indicated how good was his performance.

No matter how good a bull is, some of his sons from high-producing dams will almost certainly be as good or better than he was, virtue as always being measured by the capacity to beget high-producing daughters. There is, therefore, no commercial reason for seeking methods by which bull semen could be preserved in viable condition for decades or centuries. When, however, imaginative men start to think about the evolutionary future of man they would be liable to seize on the potentialities of human artificial insemination if long-term storage of active sperm were possible. As far as I can find from standard sources it is only with bull semen that the full viability of deep-frozen spermatozoa has been established. With horses, sheep, and poultry it has not proved practical and no extensive tests for the viability of human sperm after freezing have been reported. A few years ago a famous American geneticist, H. J. Muller, caused a stir by suggesting that the possibility of using the semen of outstanding men for artificial insemination should be seriously considered. The socially desirable qualities of men are so diverse that if one uniquely gifted individual could pass on his particular gift to, say, 50 per cent of his offspring, there could well be justification for not only using him as a donor for artificial insemination, but also for storing ampoules of his semen in liquid nitrogen to be used with suitable recipients in future generations. Muller died in 1967 and his idea does not seem likely to be brought into practice in any foreseeable future.

Even in academic circles, great achievement is not always correlated with great intelligence, nor is great intelligence regularly transmissible to children. In a long-term study of the future careers of gifted young people the results can be summarized by saying that the subjects married spouses of higher IQ than average but not as high as their own, and that their children had also a relatively high IQ but there was a wide scatter and only a small proportion would reach the intellectual level of the 'index' parents. Admittedly there are some famous upper middle-class intellectual families in England which have gone on producing highly distinguished men and women for generations. Of course, inheritance, often from both sides, has played a part but so have the home and educational environment, opportunity to excel, and the tradition of the clan.

Mullerian eugenics is only a fantasy for the foreseeable future. It would be anathema to any democracy or any political system that claimed to be a democracy, and to every man in power who had doubts of his own intrinsic quality. Yet, amongst men's dreams of human betterment, it is probably the most soundly based of them all. In some brave new world, controlled by an intellectual élite that had in some way been able to avoid the corruption of power, it could become necessary that the quality of that élite should be maintained. With sex firmly dissociated from reproduction and an intense group feeling within the élite, I can see that with a thousand more years of knowledge about human genetics, the Mullerian ethic might become a cultural imperative—but only within a ruling élite.

CONTROL OF THE SEX OF OFFSPRING

If population control ever becomes a reality and families are nominally limited to two children there would undoubtedly be a demand from some families for one of each, one boy and one girl, if there were ways of ensuring this. Even now, most of us know at least one family where a sequence of girls has gone further than would be expected from that particular couple! The general opinion of demographers is that ability to predetermine sex of desired offspring would initially at least produce a significant increase in the proportion of males which could eventually be socially disastrous. All experience indicates, however, that if a short-term benefit is available, most people will take it with complete disregard for long-term results.

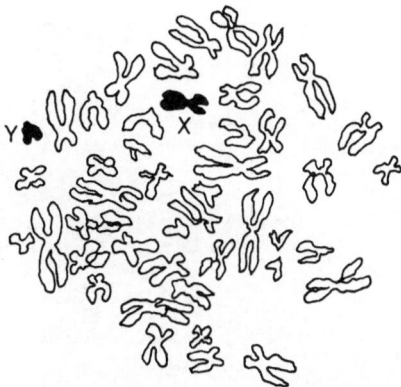

FIG. 14. Outlines of the 46 human chromosomes from a male. X and Y chromosomes are shown in black.

Sex is determined by which type of spermatozoon fertilizes the ovum. Both male and female sex cells have the half number of chromosomes (23) as compared to the full (diploid) complement (46) of a somatic cell and each has only one sex chromosome. Every ovum has an X chromosome, half the spermatozoa have X, half have Y. When fertilization takes place we have only two normal possibilities.

Sperm 22+Y and ovum 22+X gives 44+XY (male)
Sperm 22+X and ovum 22+X gives 44+XX (female).

To produce a male infant at will, it would be necessary to ensure that a 22+Y sperm was successful in fertilizing the ovum. In practice this would mean separating the two types of spermatozoa in a sample of semen, or alternatively finding some way to inactivate the female-producing (22+X) sperm while leaving the male-producers (22+Y) fully active. There have been various suggestions but none of them could really be investigated until early in 1970. Now a wholly unexpected discovery has changed the whole situation.

It is a common manœuvre in cytological laboratories to use fluorescent dyes for various types of specialized staining. For instance, if one wants to know which cell has a certain immune character, it is often possible to link a fluorescent dye to a purified antibody corresponding to the cellular antigen. Properly handled,

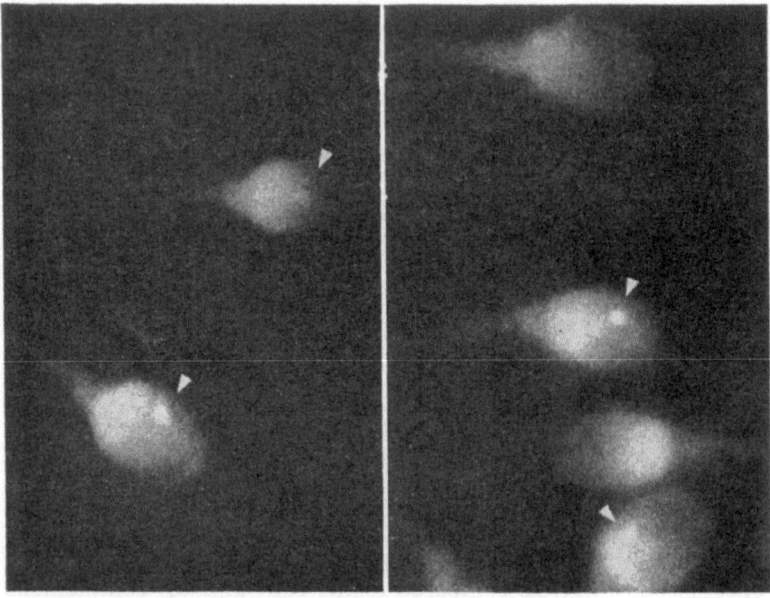

FIG. 15. Spermatozoa showing fluorescent staining of the Y region
(×4,550 approx.) (*Nature*, 1970).

that fluorescent antibody becomes, as it were, a dye capable of staining only cells with the antigen we are looking for. Examined with ultra-violet light the stained cells show a bright fluorescence which makes it possible to pick them out against a large background of dark unstained cells. Someone looking at spread-out chromosomes in this fashion found to her surprise that one chromosome developed a bright glow at one end which had nothing whatever to do with the real purpose of her experiment. It soon became clear that the fluorescent chemical being used, quinacrine, had this queer capacity to stain only one segment of one chromosome of the 46 and that the Y chromosome—the male-producer. There was even better news to follow when it was found that spermatozoa stained with quinacrine showed about 50 per cent with a small much brighter spot in the head region. No one has any doubt that this bright spot is the Y chromosome and that spermatozoa showing it would produce males while those without it would beget females.

Staining with quinacrine almost certainly kills the spermatozoon but the potential of the method is obvious. It is now possible to try all sorts of ways of separating X from Y spermatozoa, e.g., subjecting them to filtration through columns of the standard biochemical types or applying electric currents to make one sort move faster than the other. When the experiment is finished and there are two samples of sperm to be compared, it is no longer necessary to use each sample for the fertilization of large numbers of female mice, all at an appropriately receptive stage. Now any type of semen, including human, can be used and the result assessed by simple staining with quinacrine. If both samples have 50 per cent of each, obviously no separation has been obtained but if A shows 95 per cent of Y, and B shows only 20 per cent of Y, the experimenter is well on the way and before long we may find a new variant of AIH (artificial insemination—husband) with semen treated in such a fashion that it contains 99 per cent of male-producing sperm.

It is possible, in principle, but I think most obstetricians would agree that any method powerful enough to give a 99 per cent separation would be dangerously prone to damage the genetic quality of the sperm. It might be very hard to prove that this was the case but I think the possibility would in itself be enough to inhibit the use of the method. There is a random likelihood of genetic damage in something around 1 per cent of normal human pregnancies and few people would be willing to accept any significant rise in that rate. And unless human nature changes, *any* genetic damage in the offspring of a contrived insemination would almost certainly become a basis for legal action against the obstetrician concerned. Application of similar principles to domestic animals or birds would be a natural extension of artificial insemination and might have important commercial advantages—but that is not our theme.

SOMATIC CELLS

In moving to somatic cells the first point to be emphasized is that in man, all somatic cells have the full complement of 46 chromosomes, the sex chromosomes being XX in females, XY in males. In ordinary usage a somatic cell is any cell present in the general tissues of an animal but it is equally applicable to embryonic cells in their prenatal developmental stages.

Modern work on cytology (or cell science) is rather largely concerned with the behaviour of cells in the early stages of the
developing embryo on the one hand and with the phenomena
shown by cells which can be persuaded to grow outside the body in
test-tubes or more elaborate containers by the techniques of tissue
culture. For work with early embryos, laboratory animals, particularly mice, must be used but tissue cultures can now be readily
established with a variety of human cells—and, of course, with
cells from any other species of animal. For the study of fundamental biology all mammals are more or less equivalent and for most
academic purposes a mouse is as good as a man. Serious study of
cells and of embryonic development started with cold-blooded
animals simply because there was no need for incubators and
heated microscope stages to study them. Sea-urchin eggs and
frog embryos were the classical objects and much of the work
with mammalian cells has followed the pattern laid down in
the late nineteenth century with developing tadpoles and sea-
urchins.

There are still some important experiments, however, which can
only be done successfully with frog embryos, yet must be referred
to because of claims that they may be relevant in the human
biology of the future. For the most part, however, we shall not
stray far from mammalian cells.

First, one or two essential reminders about the nature of somatic
mammalian cells. A cell is a living unit basically composed of
nucleus, cytoplasm, and cell membrane. The nucleus is the
repository of DNA and its information, bundled (in man) into 46
chromosomes which only become clearly visible in the process by
which the cell divides. The cytoplasm is what can be called the
working part of the cell where proteins are made and where most
of the chemical interchanges, the cell's metabolism, take place. Its
amount relative to the size of the nucleus varies greatly from one
type of cell to another. The third component to be mentioned is
the cell membrane, the dynamic surface layer of the cell by which
it makes contact with the rest of the world and which, as will
appear later, is vital in maintaining the individuality of the cell.
Every cell has a considerable degree of autonomy; its maintenance
and when necessary its replication, i.e., its growth and division into
two cells, are under the control of the genetic information stored
in its own nucleus. Every cell is derived from the replication of a

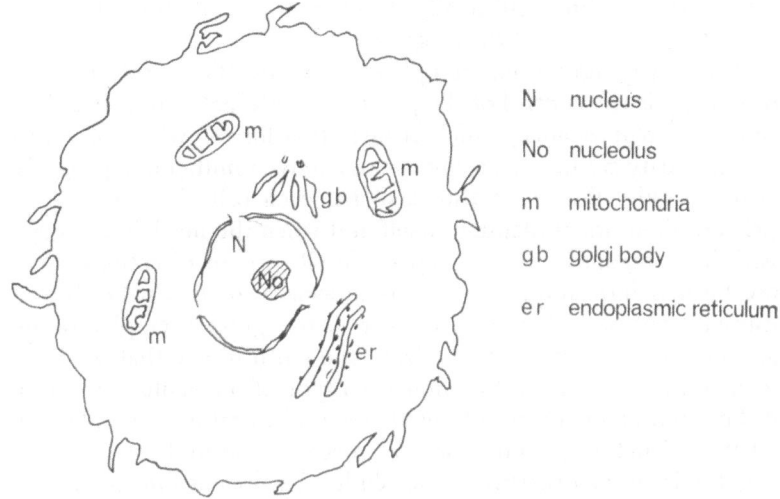

N   nucleus

No   nucleolus

m   mitochondria

gb   golgi body

er   endoplasmic reticulum

FIG. 16. Diagram of a cell.

pre-existing cell. The fertilized ovum from which each individual begins is, of course, a fusion of sperm and ovum each conveying its own 23 chromosomes, one of each pair to give the full 46 which will be characteristic of almost every somatic cell of the body. One feels that one should be saying that *all* somatic cells have 46 chromosomes but there was never a biological generalization without exceptions and some apparently normal liver cells have an extra set. The 46 chromosomes in each somatic cell presumably contain the same information as there was in the zygote and one of the main things we have to discuss is how this is compatible with the immense differences in form and function of cells.

Differentiation is all-important but so also is the continuity of cellular descent. I have found it enlightening at times to look at an individual, at oneself particularly, as a four-dimensional clone of cells. A clone from the Greek meaning, a branching twig, is used for any set of descendant cells arising from a single initiating cell. A man's life, then, is a four-dimensional clone in time which, if one pictures it in two dimensions, one of them time, gives something shaped like a rocket, starting from the minute granule of the zygote, proliferating smoothly to reach a standard size and number at twenty years and past fifty, beginning to show irregularities and terminated cell lines, till finally the clone frays out and a few days after death the last cell disintegrates.

Necessarily, no cell has complete autonomy. The greatest riddle of biology is the control of the process of differentiation, organization, and maintenance, which ensures that for the whole of youth and maturity we have a seeing eye, an active mind, and a properly shaped ankle. For these things to be, each cell must be appropriately sited, must maintain itself and when the need arises, cope with local regeneration and repair. In all sorts of directions there are limited indications of how some aspects of this over-all and mutual control is handled. Cancer is the great exemplar of its absence. Perhaps it is not far from the truth to say that we have gained a fair understanding how each type of molecule found in a cell or an organism comes to be there and in a rather general sense what its function is. There is, too, a reasonable understanding of *why* the internal structure of the cell has its standard form. On the other hand there is hardly the beginning of an approach as to *how* the molecules are organized into structures within the cells and how cells come to take the right place and the right form at the right time to allow proper development of the organism. Much play is being made at the present time with the phrase self-assembly.

It is now dogma that the sequence of amino acids in the one-dimensional polypeptide chain coming off the cellular assembly line, is sufficient to determine the exact three-dimensional configuration the chain will take to produce a functional protein. At the next higher level it is suggested that the coat protein of a virus is so structured that the only way a group of the molecules can make a stable aggregate is to create a geometrically symmetrical shell, often an icosahedron, within which the other requirements for the virus can be neatly packed.

Such self-assembly processes must be important and it may be that it will never be possible to go beyond explanations in that general form. After all, unless an organism *can* assemble itself correctly it will not survive. But it is hardly a satisfying interpretation. To me at least, nothing gives a greater sense of intellectual impotence than the realization that every cell in our bodies has a nucleus which by every rule of genetic logic contains potentially as much information as any other—and that there is no master cell nor any other fount of information in the body. It may be only a human weakness that this should seem to be extraordinary and inexplicable. There is equally no autocrat, no central control in the beehive, the ant-nest, or the termite mound.

TISSUE CULTURE

This is just a preliminary to speaking of tissue culture. Many different types of body cell will, given the right conditions, multiply freely outside the body. The physical conditions must be right, temperature, an appropriate solution which, if the conditions are to be chemically defined may require seventy or more ingredients though, more often, some biological mixtures like foetal calf serum or chick embryo extract are more convenient to use. Most experts in tissue culture have, in addition, their own tricks to get cultures started, particularly when it is required to initiate a pure clone culture from a single cell. With good modern technique, cells in tissue culture are essentially similar to the body cells they spring from in having the same complement of chromosomes and the same immunological character. There are now many examples where cells taken from some tissue in an embryo can continue growing in tissue culture and change (differentiate) from a primitive undifferentiated cell to something with specific structure and function such as a muscle cell.

But a tissue culture is not part of a functioning organism, it is not a tissue and its limitations for providing models of bodily function will always be obvious, though the enthusiast may be right that there is no limit to the approach to normality that will be eventually achieved. Some of the difficulties may be mentioned briefly.

In the first place the cells in a good tissue culture are multiplying freely since, in general, that is what the experimenter is looking for. There are, however, only a few places in a grown animal where cells are multiplying at the sort of rate one looks for in tissue culture. Bone marrow, thymus, and intestinal lining are the important sites. As might be expected, it is much simpler to initiate tissue cultures from cells that are already growing rapidly, such as malignant cells from an established tumour or cells from a young embryo than from normal adult cells.

Second, there is a mutual assistance effect in tissue culture. If one has a good actively growing cell culture in solution A and transfers a single cell to a new container of the same solution it will fail to grow. To start a new clone from a single cell, special arrangements to provide products of cell growth are necessary. In due course these will no doubt be identified but for the present one can merely speak of the need for products diffusing from adjacent cells.

Possibly related in some way to this phenomenon is the finding that human cells in tissue culture cannot survive and continue to multiply under what appear to be optimal conditions for more than approximately fifty generations. This limit of fifty generations is called after the cytologist who discovered it, the Hayflick limit. Those fifty generations are exceeded only if a rather gross form of mutation occurs with alteration of the chromosome number. There is still some reasonable doubt about the significance of the Hayflick limit. It is still possible that it has no significant bearing on what happens in the body, perhaps because it is a mere indication of some unrecognized inadequacy of tissue culture techniques. If it is also a manifestation of what happens to cell lines in the body it could have important implications for the process of ageing.

There is no doubt, however, about the fact that under certain circumstances, presumably as a result of a mutation, a tissue culture begins to grow much more freely and a new cell line takes command nearly always showing an abnormal set of chromosomes. If this capacity for free growth takes place in a tissue culture derived from a closely inbred strain of mice it is possible to test the rapidly growing cells for their capacity to produce a tumour when injected into mice of the same strain. A fair proportion can in this way be shown to have undergone transformation to cancer cells. It is by no means axiomatic that the capacity to grow without limit in tissue culture can be equated with malignancy. What can be said is that once transformation to free growth has occurred, other mutations occur readily and amongst these some will overgrow the standard cell form and some, when transferred to the original host, will produce evidence of malignancy. In some experiments which provoked a considerable controversy this was done using human cell cultures transferred to patients with inoperable cancer. Much more satisfactory studies have been made with cells from mice. In one famous experiment two lines of cell transfers were established in tissue culture from the same initial cell. After a long series of transfers, cells from both lines were inoculated into mice of the same strain as provided the initial cell. One line gave a typical malignant tumour, a sarcoma that went on to kill the host, the other gave an initial tumour-like proliferation that subsequently disappeared, presumably being overcome by the animal's own immune response. The experiment underlines two important points. The first is that in every population of growing cells there is a competition for survival. A rapidly growing mutant will outgrow and replace unmutated cells. The second is that mutation to malignancy is not a standardized process. Mutations are rare, random, and diverse, and the eventual mutant types which come to dominate two cultures started from the same source may differ in many respects including their capacity to produce cancer in the parent strain. It is worth underlining, too, that no mutation will become evident unless the existing conditions or special conditions arranged by the experimenter provide a special advantage for proliferation and survival to the mutant form. That sentence states an absolutely crucial requirement for the understanding of everything that has to do with mutation in somatic (body) cells and it is particularly relevant to the understanding of cancer. We shall return again to this when we deal with cancer and its problems for the future, in Chapter 7.

CELLULAR POTENTIALITIES

I have already said that according to the logic of genetics every single cell in an organism possesses the full potentiality of the zygote (fertilized ovum) from which the whole organism developed. In principle this implies that if we could provide the right conditions for its development, any cell in the body could grow into a complete human being, an identical twin, as it were, of the person who provided the somatic cell. No one has even approached this experimentally in any animal but in plants it has actually been accomplished. A tissue culture started from cells of the growing shoot on a tobacco plant can be sorted out into single cells and with appropriate coaxing, one of those cells will develop into a complete tobacco plant, roots, leaves, flowers, and all. Plants, however, are not animals and the dictum that every somatic cell in an animal equally contains the same complete genetic information, rests on logic rather than experiment. Human somatic cells divide like all typical cells in such a fashion that the structure of the chromosomes (and the information they carry) is exactly duplicated at every division. Once egg and sperm have united to give the full 46 chromosomes in the zygote, the whole sequence of their descendant cells, with only a few unimportant exceptions will have the same 46 chromosomes and the same fund of potential information. It is obvious, however, that once an organism starts to take form and relegate different functions to different organs, all cells cannot remain alike. In each organ the cells must concentrate on developing those qualities and only those qualities that are needed in that particular organ. This holds also in regard to the functions of cleaning up and repair that must follow injury or infection of a local region of the body. It would be most inconvenient and alarming if after any minor cut or abrasion a baby started to develop on the region. There *are* primitive animals which behave in this fashion, the freshwater *Hydra* for example, and even within the vertebrates, even in man, there are accidental or experimental occurrences which underline the wide potentiality, the toti-potency, of all somatic cells. Here is another region where the speculators, the enthusiasts, the apostles of progress have been looking for potential improvement of the human lot. Nature using only the random shuffle of the genes occasionally produces men of the quality of Newton, Descartes, Pascal, Goethe, Shakespeare—but only once in a million or a hundred million births. How wonderful, say the dreamers, if in ten or twenty years' time the man who, shall we say, brings durable peace and disarmament to the world could provide a tissue culture of his cells to be stored in liquid nitrogen. Every five years one of those cells could be stimulated to re-mobilize its potentialities and take on the character of the zygote it came from. Some young woman will doubtless be proud to have the zygote implanted in her uterus and become its mother. So, the dream goes, we can ensure the world of a series of men— identical twins of the great man—who, properly educated in the contemporary scene, will grow up with the same political skills but each with a new and up-to-date social background. It sounds and probably is ridiculous but it is worth looking closely at the material on which such dreams might be based.

First we have the Briggs and King experiment with frog embryos.

Suppose one takes newly fertilized frog spawn from two closely related but easily distinguished species *A* and *B*. By the use of micro-manipulators with an array of tiny knives, needles, suction tubes, and injection tubes it is possible to place an *A* frog egg on the stage of a microscope and extract its nucleus. The same can be done with a *B* egg. Then the *A* nucleus can be placed in the cytoplasm of the *B* egg and vice versa. If one carries out several dozen of such reciprocal transfers, a proportion of the transposed cells will develop and a few will even go right through to adult frogs. In all, the frog will have the colour markings and other qualities of the frog which provided the nucleus.

This is just what one would expect if the experiment could be done at all. After all, one assumes that all the essential information must be in the zygote nucleus. It merely represents a necessary preliminary to an account of Briggs and King's experiment in 1952, and elaborations of it since. Their experiment was to remove the nucleus from a freshly fertilized frog ovum and replace it with a nucleus from tissues of frog embryos at various stages of development. At the so-called blastula stage, i.e., when the primary ball of dividing cells develops a central cavity, a nucleus from any of these 40–60 cells can replace the original nucleus of the zygote and allow development to a considerable degree, sometimes as far as metamorphosis to the adult. With cells from older embryos the experiment failed but there have been more recent claims to have obtained normal embryos from nuclei of well-advanced cells of the intestinal region.

This suggests strongly that, provided the increasing technical difficulties of doing the experiment are overcome, the nucleus continues to carry the full content of information through many divisions and can still manifest it when placed in the appropriate environment of the zygote cytoplasm.

In a sense this does not tell us much more than the famous experiment of Hans Driech which created a sensation amongst the philosophers in the 1890s. A fertilized sea-urchin egg is a globe which divides into 2, then by a segmentation at right angles into

4 and then via 8, 16, etc., to the blastula stage and eventually the active larva. If after the first of these primary segmentations the two resulting cells are gently separated each develops into a somewhat smaller but perfectly normal sea-urchin larva. Normally the nuclei of the first division would work in concert to produce what was allotted to them and their descendant cells in the construction of the predestined single individual. When, however, they were separated by the experimenter's whim, each showed the full capacity to create a whole organism.

At the human level this happens with every pair of identical twins. Sometimes the process goes farther and it is accepted that the Dionne quintuplets arose from a single fertilization. Three of the second generation nuclei and two of the third generation manifested their capacity to shape five identical human beings. Most readers will remember Aldous Huxley's Bokhanowsky groups of deltas in *Brave New World*, produced by splitting the ovum *ad lib* and culturing each segment separately. They were quite remarkably convenient for various types of group industrial activity!

There are many other experiments which might be cited to indicate the intrinsic potentialities of all the nuclei in that four-dimensional clone that is a human or another mammalian life. Two only can be mentioned here because, again, there are just conceivably human implications that arise from them. The first concerns Mintz's allophenic mice. It is almost exactly the converse of Driesch's sea-urchin eggs and the Dionne quins. Instead of splitting one predestined embryo to make two or five, Mintz takes two predestined embryos and fuses them to produce in due course, what she calls an allophenic mouse—a mouse with literally four parents.

As in all the experiments I have described, there are manifold technical difficulties to be overcome but when we are interested only in the result and its significance, the technical side can be forgotten. In outline, Beatrice Mintz takes a young embryo of strain A from the uterus of its mother and another of strain B from the uterus of *its* mother. The two embryos (both at the blastocyst stage) are freed of surrounding material and pressed gently together. Within twenty-four hours the cells come together in essentially random fashion and sort themselves out

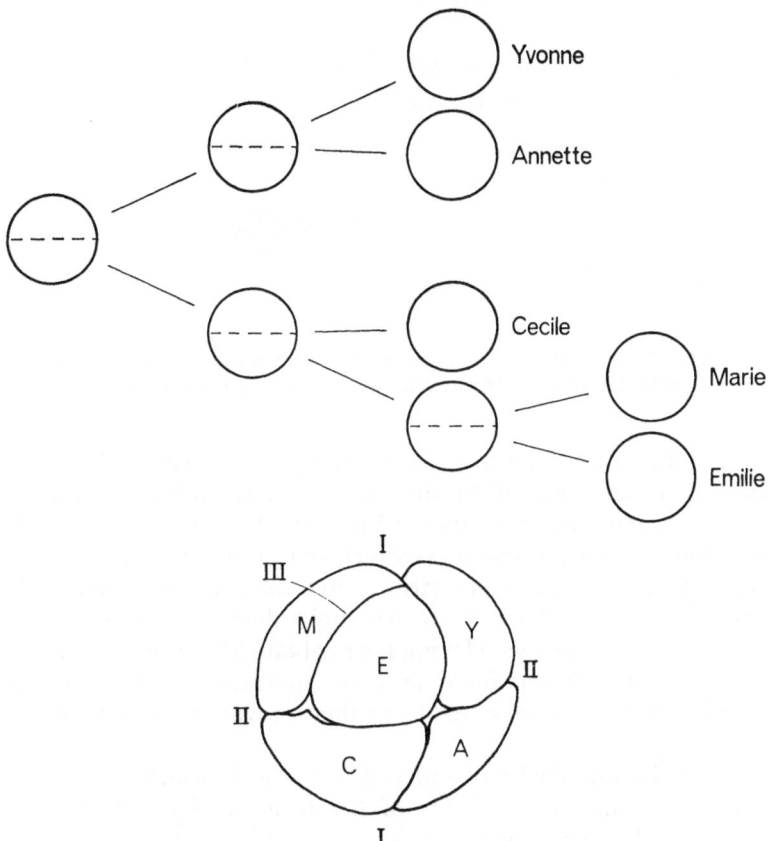

FIG. 17. The Dionne quintuplets (after Newman).

to make a single larger blastocyst. This, still a very small speck of living material, is now gently transferred to the uterus of a foster mother of strain *C*. If all goes well, mouse *C* will give birth in due course to baby mice corresponding to some or all of the fused embryos that were surgically inserted into her uturus.

The mice are healthy functional mice but they can show the curious character of their origin in various ways. If an *A* female is fused with a male *B*, a problem is presented which can be solved in various ways, usually by the almost complete dominance of one

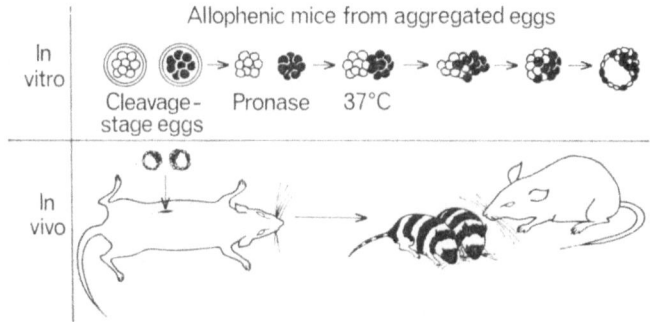

FIG. 18. A diagram showing the Mintz technique for producing allophenic mice (*Proc. Nat. Acad. Sci.* **58** (1967), 344).

sex. More striking is the range of skin patterns when *A* is white and *B* is black. Some of the allophenes are striped black and white and, of course, they are called zebra mice. Even the most sharply bi-colour mice have markings which only roughly correspond to alternate black and white stripes and most of the group will approach one or other of the parental colours with only poorly differentiated markings. Having heard about zebra mice, one tends to be slightly disappointed at their appearance but when the allophenes are looked at in detail they provide some fascinating stories.

To an immunologist like myself, the way in which single cells and patches of cells of *A* and of *B* can be fused together into a mosaic and function perfectly is of special interest. Anyone with even a passing interest in the stories of kidney and heart transplants that were the popular scientific sensation of the 1960s, knows that the body normally rejects any grafted tissues that are not its own. Plastic surgeons can repair a disastrously mutilated face with skin grafts from any other part of the patient's body but not from another donor. The only exception is when the donor is an identical twin. In medical investigations where it is absolutely essential to be certain that two people are in fact identical twins the final test is to remove two equal-sized circles of skin from each and transplant them reciprocally. If *A*'s piece of skin heals normally and looks healthy on *B*, and *B*'s piece does the same on *A*, then *A* and *B* are identical twins. The first kidney transplants were in fact done only when the patient with serious kidney disease had

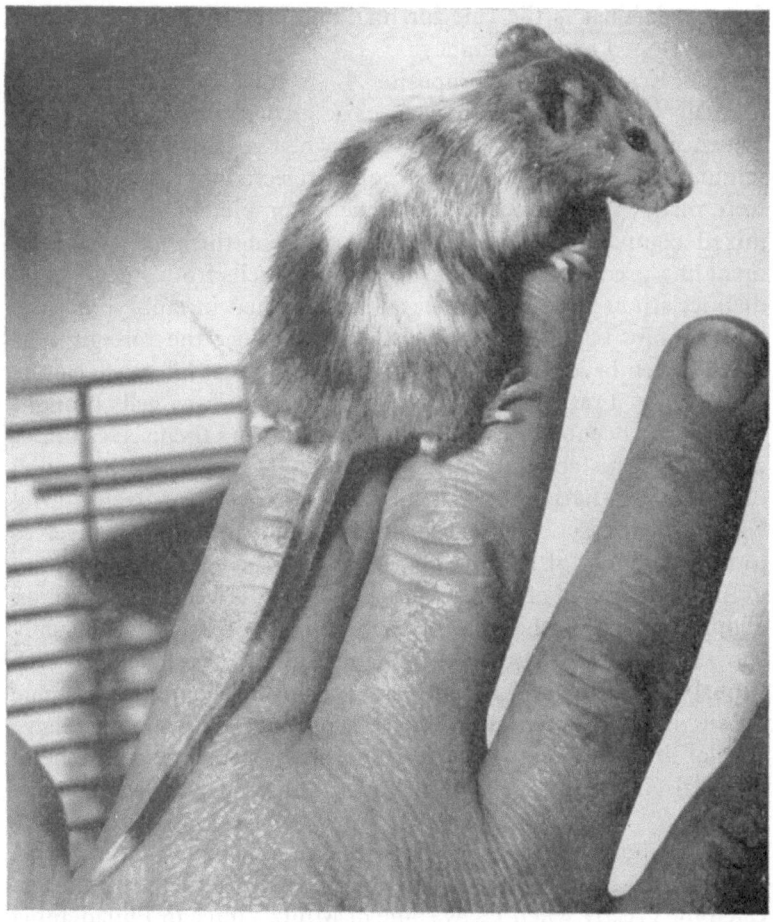

FIG. 19. A photograph of an allophenic (zebra) mouse.
(By courtesy of Dr Margaret Holmes, The Walter and Eliza Hall
Institute.)

an identical twin willing to donate a kidney. Most kidneys for
transplantation nowadays come from persons who have died
suddenly from road accidents or other cause, and if they are to be
accepted, an elaborate regime of immunosuppressive drugs is
necessary to block the rejection response. Foreign cells in the body
are recognized as foreign, provoke an immune response and are

destroyed. That is the rule for man and any other mammal that has developed beyond infancy.

In Beatrice Mintz's composite $A+B$ mice there will be two mutually foreign types of cell in close association yet there is no evidence of any incompatibility even when A and B are far apart immunologically and would be rapidly rejected if cross skin grafts were made; the composite allophene is completely tolerant of its mixed components. These results represent the final establishment of a prediction I made in 1949 that if cells from a genetically distinct strain were implanted and established in embryonic life, no antibody response should be made against the foreign cells when the embryo reached adult life. This mutual tolerance can be looked at as a rather specialized example of the way cells brought together early enough can in some fashion bring themselves under a mutually satisfactory control. There is a lot to suggest that much of the process by which a functional body constructs itself during embryonic life depends on the ability of cells to adjust themselves to the proximity of the cell that *happens* to be adjacent.

Another feature of general interest to be derived from work on allophenic mice is that appropriate methods of study will usually show that every tissue represents a mosaic of A and B cells. This probably has the implication that at least up to the blastocyst stage no single cell is predestined for the production of any exclusive type of differentiated cell. The fate of its descendants will depend on local circumstances as they emerge in the course of development.

At this point it is worth reverting for a moment to the story I told in Chapter 1, of fleece mosaics in Australian sheep. It interested me greatly when I saw some of Mintz's mice in Philadelphia that the distribution of the white bands on an otherwise dark-coloured animal had very much the same form as the vertical patches of long wool on the mosaic sheep.

In many ways the situation of a sheep embryo with one out of four cells carrying a long-wool mutation is closely analogous to that of a 'white' mouse embryo with which a 'black' embryo has been fused artificially. There is much to be learnt from an analysis and comparison of the spatial distribution of long hair in these sheep and of black and white regions in Mintz's allophenic mice. In both we have certain cell lines founded very early in embryonic life which have to compete for final expression in the animal with other lines. In the early stage each line has the full potentiality of producing every other type of cell—Mintz's experiments even indicate that the possibility of becoming germ cells is also included in those potentialities. In the sheep, if Fraser and Short's interpretation is correct, one can deduce that at least up to the 16- or 32-cell stage, every cell has some future responsibility for the nature of the wool that the animal will produce.

CELL FUSION

There is one final approach to the brave new world of genetic manipulation, nuclear fusion of somatic cells. This is based on the Japanese discovery that tissue culture cells could be fused by treatment with Sendai virus which belongs to the influenza group of viruses (Myxovirus). Heat-killed virus acts almost as well as living. The surface of an animal cell, whether in the body or in tissue culture, provides a very important boundary with highly significant functions. In fact almost the whole individuality of a cell seems to reside in its surface. To take one or two examples we can start with the entry of polio virus into a cell. Polio virus will readily infect and multiply within monkey kidney cells but it has no capacity to infect chick embryo cells. There is quite an elaborate interaction between the cell surface components and the polio virus before entrance is effected into a susceptible monkey cell. When the surface components are inappropriate as in chicken or hamster cells the process fails, yet in Enders's laboratory in 1967 it was shown that treatment of either type of cell with Sendai virus would let some polio virus slip into the substance of the cell without being held up by the cell surface. Once there, it multiplied freely.

More immediately relevant is the possibility of fusing two different cell types so that in effect nucleus A and nucleus B inhabit a common pool of cytoplasm. Even when the two cells are as remote as a human cancer cell and a fowl red blood cell (which, unlike mammalian red cells, has a nucleus) the two nuclei get on happily together. The rather shrunken red cell nucleus actually enlarges and gives evidence of functional activity it would never normally possess. In other experiments in which mixed mouse and human cells are used, two distinct nuclei can divide in the same cytoplasm in essentially normal fashion. If the divisions can be synchronized the two nuclei (man and mouse) may join forces and produce a single nucleus with initially about 86 chromosomes and subsequently continue dividing. The division is not done expertly and the number of chromosomes falls usually to something around forty after some generations. The nuclear division may be done rather ineffectively but the fact that it is done at all gives a surprising indication of how made to a pattern the mammalian mechanisms of nuclear division must be and how important for the individuality of the cell is the elaborately interrelated mosaic of functional molecules on its surface.

In June 1969, I was fortunate enough to be staying at the Villa Serbelloni on Lake Como when a small technical conference met to discuss phenomena of this sort in both animals and plants. I was invited to sit in at the meetings and found them full of interest and with a distinct flavour of science fiction. It was accepted by all, that joint mouse–man cells with composite nuclei could be produced. No one suggested that a mouse–man hybrid could be grown from one of those cells but the botanists were excited about what might develop if similar cell fusion could be brought about in plant cells.

On a previous page I have mentioned how, for some plant species at least, it is possible to derive a complete plant from a single cell growing in plant tissue culture. I pointed out then, that this was the ultimate proof that a single somatic cell of the plant carries all the information needed to build the whole organism. What the botanists had in mind was the possibility of an incomparably wide range of hybridizations if a means could be found to fuse somatic cells of almost unrelated species and persuade such unnatural hybrids to develop into complete plants. If cells of man and fowl or man and mouse can produce composite cells which can multiply in tissue culture, why should not a cell of a high-bearing rice hybridize with a desirable strain of sweet potato? And if a tobacco or begonia single cell can produce a complete plant of its proper type, why should not the hybrid cell produce a plant with the virtues of both its parents? So far as I am aware, no such artificial fusion of plant cells has yet produced a complete composite plant but I know that a variety of possible approaches is being explored.

4

HUMAN APPLICATIONS
FOR THE 'NEW' BIOLOGY

This is the century, we are told, in which innovation and scientific-technological advance—progress in other words—should be able to produce anything within the limits of what is physically possible in principle. We have only to want it sufficiently and to pay the price and we can have it. If rocks from the moon can be brought to Houston, why should we not be able to apply molecular biology, cytology, and the rest, to cure what is now incurable? In this chapter I want to look primarily at the potential applications of molecular biology to human affairs and later at one or two of the suggestions that are current for other revolutionary developments.

MOLECULAR BIOLOGY

I have more than once expressed the opinion that so far there has been no human benefit whatever from all that has been learnt of molecular biology. I doubt if any other biological scientist has been quite so blunt in public but a few eminent biochemists have agreed with me in private.

The ostensible justification for medical research is for the improvement of human health and medical care. By Nobel's will, Nobel prizes were to be given to those who 'during the preceding year shall have conferred the greatest benefit on mankind'. Since 1957, eighteen chemists and biochemists have shared eight Nobel prizes for work on proteins, nucleic acids, and their significance and there can be little doubt that apart from clinical research, with its special human responsibilities, a larger number of highly distinguished workers and more money were applied to molecular biology in the last five years than to any other biological field. Molecular biology is undoubtedly the fashionable science, the one in which reputations are made, whose successes are applauded by presidents and royalty and from which the public, guided mainly by what scientists are said to have told journalists, expects some dramatic human dividends in the future.

Genetic engineering

The expected benefit is felt to concern those conditions of disease or disability which are ascribed to faulty inheritance or to genetic change in cells which have taken on disease-producing (pathogenic) activity. If we can synthesize a gene of the 'right' type, why not use it to replace the bad gene more or less in the way that we can use an accident victim's healthy kidney to replace a diseased one? A boy suffers from the bleeding disease haemophilia because a mutation in one of his ancestors has given him a faulty gene which fails to make one of the factors needed to allow blood to clot normally. He can nowadays be kept free from major haemorrhages by appropriate use of very expensive products extracted from normal human blood. Surely it would be more satisfactory for everybody if the right gene could be inserted into his X chromosome—this being one of the few human genetic conditions in which we know which of the 46 chromosomes carries the faulty gene. In another field most biologists agree that subject to minor qualifications a cancer is a mass of cells derived from a single ancestral cell which became abnormal as a result of a change in one or more genes. All the descendant cells which make up the cancer, carry the same unfortunate genes. To the unsophisticated layman there seems an obvious opportunity to change the character of the pathogenic cells preferably well before the cancer grows sufficiently to cause trouble.

Everybody with a reasonable knowledge of biology and medicine is well aware that these things cannot be done now. To my mind, however, far too many take the point of view in public that the latest achievement in molecular biology is a giant step forward toward achieving control of something of importance to medicine. It may not come in our lifetime but so-and-so's achievement shows that it is on the way.

I was very unhappy to see the words that American newspapers put into the mouths of Kornberg and others when his synthesis of DNA was announced in December 1967. The term synthesis is in one sense correct but it was not a synthesis in the chemist's sense but a brilliantly controlled imitation of nature's method, using enzymes and other biologically produced components to do so.

Kornberg produced large amounts of the DNA of a virus, a bacteriophage, 'in the test tube'. The bacterial virus which he used is much simpler than the bacterium at whose expense it grows, yet as I have indicated earlier it has its own 'blueprint', its DNA, which by seizing, as it were, its host's synthetic machinery, can persuade or command it to make the protein shell and tail of the virus, instead of material proper to the bacterium. Kornberg's achievement was undoubtedly a biochemical *tour de force* but it hardly deserved what the President or his speech-writer thought appropriate for the occasion—that it 'opens a wide door to new discoveries in fighting disease and building healthier lives for mankind . . . The first step towards the future control of certain types of cancer.' Kornberg, who shared a Nobel prize in 1959 for his work in showing how DNA multiplied, made, according to the Press, a suggestion that it might be possible to extend such results to another sort of virus and come closer to the possibility of genetic engineering. There is, for instance, a virus which under special conditions can produce a variety of cancers in baby mice or hamsters. It is known as polyoma virus and it has been very extensively studied. I shall have a good deal to say about it in Chapter 7, but here all that need be said is that it has DNA for its blueprint and can sometimes change mammalian cells genetically without destroying them. If we know what sort of a gene is needed, then in Kornberg's words: 'It may be possible then to attach a gene to a harmless viral DNA and use this virus as a vehicle for delivering a gene to the cells of a patient suffering from a heredi-tary defect and thereby cure him.' This is one of the more specific suggestions as to how molecular biology might be channelled to human benefit. It will later serve as a text for discussion.

Another way of handling the same problem of replacing a faulty gene that was responsible for a patient's disability, with a good gene has been sketched by Tatum. His suggestion was that the good gene might be incorporated into a tissue culture of the patient's own cells. When a cell into which the synthetic gene had been incorporated and was functioning, was recognized it would serve as ancestral cell for a very large family of descendant cells to be grown in tissue culture—in the test-tube as we say, though in fact it would need to be a very complex test-tube. Once a pound or two of cells had been produced the fact that the cells were still essentially the same as other cells in the patient's body would,

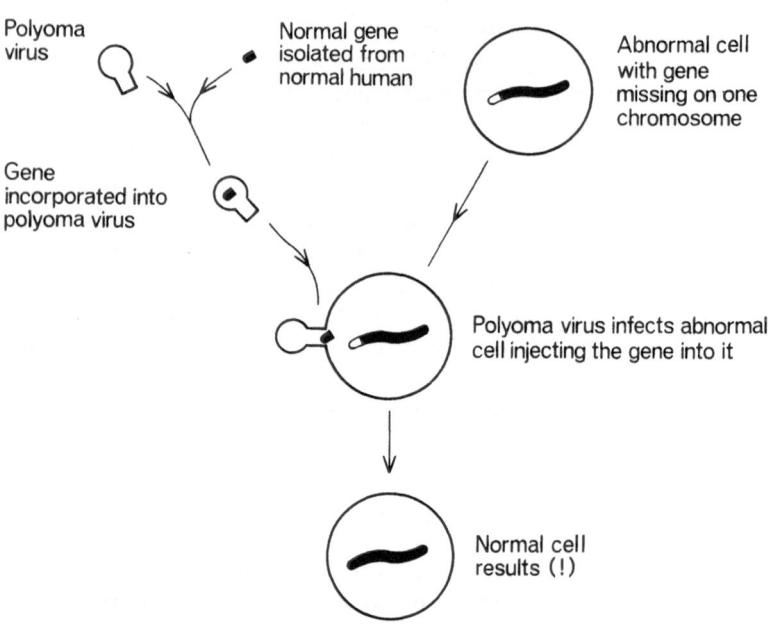

FIG. 20. A dream of genetic engineering: Kornberg's plan to replace a missing or abnormal gene.

hopefully, allow them to be established in the body perhaps as a new lobe of the liver. In principle, and if all went well, that pound of remoulded cells should produce enough of the missing component to bring the clinical disability under control.

These are the only two suggestions that I have seen made by responsible people about eventual applications of modern achievements in molecular biology to human benefit. According to my interpretation of their remarks neither Kornberg nor Tatum had any serious thought that wholly synthetic genes should ever be used for such purposes. What they were envisaging in principle was that in due course it could become possible to extract from normal human cells the sequence of DNA that was missing from or wrongly made in the patient. Once isolated these could be used as the pattern, the template, for the synthesis by bacterial enzymes of numerous replicas of itself. This is acceptable as a possibility of the foreseeable future. The next step would be the crucial and probably impossible one, to incorporate the gene into the genetic mechanism of a suitable virus vehicle in such a fashion that the virus in its turn will transfer the gene it is carrying to cells throughout the body and in the process precisely replace the faulty gene with the right one. I should be willing to state in any company that the chance of doing this will remain infinitely small to the last syllable of recorded time.

The approach via transforming a tissue culture of the patient's own cells with its more modest objective of producing a mere sufficiency of some enzyme or metabolite that is lacking, comes closer to realism. It is conceivable that with a very large population of cells exposed to the right gene a tiny fraction might incorporate it. If they or one of them could be recognized and isolated from the rest so that a pure tissue culture of 'restored' cells could be built up there could be some justification for testing them in selected conditions. The very real risk that the cells would be malignant after such manipulations would probably always be an effective deterrent to their use.

The two hypothetical procedures I have cited really involve work at the cellular genetic level rather than at the molecular one but it would still be fair to claim that the experience gained at the molecular level would certainly be necessary if there was to be any chance of success from such manipulations.

I have said enough already to make it clear that even so small an agent as an RNA bacterial virus is chemically a very complex structure. At the present time it is just beyond but not very far beyond the possibility of complete interpretation in terms of structural chemistry. With the exponential increase in difficulty of chemical study with each increase in the complexity of biological organization, I feel justified in saying that at the *molecular* level significant modification of genetic structure is only conceivable in relation to viruses.

Viruses made to order

The question therefore immediately arises as to what humanly desired changes could be made by molecular-genetic manipulation of small viruses. Bacterial viruses are never thought of nowadays as possible therapeutic agents and d'Herelle's dreams of controlling cholera and dysentery by seeding village populations with phage have been forgotten for forty years. No one is likely to take a hypervirulent anti-cholera phage as an objective for molecular manipulation of bacterial viruses and one can feel even more certain that the current favourite object of academic study, the RNA coli-phages, will have no direct bearing on human affairs.

This leaves us with the animal (including human) viruses as the only material to be seriously considered for molecular manipulation. So far there has been no real approach toward modifying animal viruses in a molecularly defined fashion and in any case this will presumably have to wait until well after an RNA phage with its 3,500 nucleotide units which correspond to three distinct RNA genes, has been completely analysed. Of the animal viruses the three types of polio virus which are responsible for poliomyelitis (polio or infantile paralysis) provide the greatest potential interest. Each virus unit of a polio virus has about 6,000 units in its RNA and perhaps 6 genes. All three types of polio virus have fairly similar proportions of the four nucleotides A, G, C, and U, so that the differences in RNA structure between different types and strains are probably small.

There are potentially useful reasons for manipulating the RNA of polio viruses. Since 1960 everyone has heard of Sabin's living virus vaccine against polio. Superficially it seems absurdly simple, just a teaspoonful of fluid by mouth or on a lump of sugar, and a near certainty of complete protection against polio for life. Behind it, however, there were years of work before a satisfactorily protective vaccine was produced. Sabin-type living vaccines are selected strains of polio viruses each presumably of defined chemical pattern, which have the 'right' degree of virulence to infect the human intestine with near certainty, and never to produce central nervous system infection with paralysis. The vaccine strains were the result of rigid but basically empirical selection procedures that made use of the fact, just as relevant to a polio virus as to a bacterium on a human cell, that inheritable changes, mutations are always occurring spontaneously. The more frequently a living unit multiplies and the more of them there are, the greater will be the number and range of mutants available for selection. It was possible for Sabin to handle the enormous populations of virus units that grew in his tissue cultures, so as to select the kind he wanted without knowing anything about the chemical structures that were responsible for the virtues of the strains he chose. It is conceivable that in twenty or fifty years' time, complete chemical understanding of polio viruses, especially of their RNA

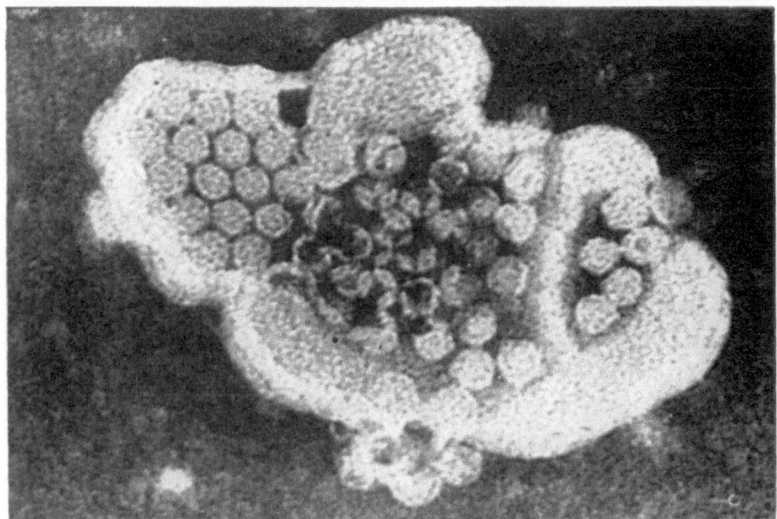

FIG. 21. An electron-micrograph of polio virus type 1 (×140,000 approx.). (By courtesy of the John Innes Institute.)

structure could help to produce better vaccines. Perhaps the one niggling doubt about the Sabin vaccine that the harmless domesticated viruses it contains might revert by mutation to virulence could be overcome if we had that knowledge.

To the medical virologist and epidemiologist there are only two qualities of polio virus that matter—virulence and antigenicity. It is rather highly probable that neither is a simple quality controlled by a single sequence in one gene. The most systematic genetic study of polio virus was concerned with a special and highly artificial study of virulence involving the use of temperature-sensitive variants (ts). A standard polio virus will grow in tissue culture at any temperature from 32 to 39 °C, but rather frequently one finds mutants which grow at 33 °C but fail to do so at 37 °C. These are ts mutants and since a monkey's temperature is something over 37 °C they are non-virulent for monkeys and presumably for man. It was found in Canberra that by treating polio viruses with a chemical (5-fluorouracil) which is an active producer of mutants, many dozens of ts mutants could be obtained. Without attempting to go into technicalities it was possible to divide these into four groups suggesting that changes on any one of four genes could produce this particular type of change. Fenner, in reviewing the results, suggested that to be fully virulent each protein must be properly constituted. Very often a single amino acid change will be sufficient to make the virus unstable at a slightly higher temperature.

It is likely to be quite fantastically difficult to map out the sequence of 6,000 nucleotide units of the polio viruses and define the four or six genes probably involved. As far as can be seen, however, no fundamental new principle needs to be discovered to make it possible. To go further and determine how the antigenic type of a virus or its virulence, its capacity to produce paralysis in man, is related to the chemical structure of its RNA and of the proteins of its coat will be very much more difficult. So far, such work has never been attempted and before going on to discuss how dangerous those studies might be, a little more needs to be said about those two qualities of antigenicity and virulence.

We say that there are three antigenic types of polio virus, Types I, II, and III. This simply means that a mild infection with Type I or administration of a Type I vaccine will immunize a child or a monkey against subsequent infection and paralysis with a Type I polio virus but not against Types II and III. The same capacity to immunize only against its own type holds equally for Type II or Type III. To vaccinate against polio we must obviously use all three types.

By virulence we mean the capacity to produce significant disease which in the case of polio virus means paralysis. Different strains of virus can differ enormously in their virulence. We can, owing to a mishap in 1956, compare two well-known strains of polio virus in regard to their virulence for children. Salk vaccine is made from virus killed by formalin. By some inadequacy of preparation, a batch of vaccine was used in which what must have been a tiny proportion of the Type I component (Strain Mahony) was still alive. Sixty-seven children were paralysed, some fatally, by their immunizing dose. At the other extreme is the Type I virus in the Sabin vaccine, selected and certified to have no capacity whatever to produce paralysis in child or monkey.

I believe that it is justifiable to say that unless something wholly unexpected arrives to short-cut procedures there is no foreseeable possibility of understanding the molecular basis of virulence and antigenicity in polio virus. Since it is the smallest and most intensively studied of the animal viruses we can extend that statement to all of them. If an ideal living virus vaccine is to be sought the only approaches are the genetic rather than the molecular level— in the same general way that Sabin developed his vaccine strain of polio.

There was a time when I was immensely interested in the genetics of influenza viruses. It was before the days of molecular biology and in the first instance my ambition was no more than to sort out how the various inheritable qualities that differentiate one strain of influenza virus from another could be expressed in the hybrids (recombinants) that I was able to obtain. It was the first such work with animal viruses and as it developed, I began to visualize a first-rate practical use for such recombination procedures. The great influenza pandemic of 1918 almost certainly represented the emergence of a new antigenic type—now called 'Swine'—of influenza A. It was associated with some 50 million deaths. Subsequent appearance of the new types A^0 ?1928–30, A^1 1946, A^2 1957, have not been so conspicuous. Although the last ('Asian 'flu') received a great deal of publicity, mortality was not exceptional. In the early 1950s, however, it seemed important to be prepared to produce large amounts of appropriate vaccine if a *new* and dangerous antigenic type of influenza were to arise.

No vaccine can be made in large amount as soon as a new virus is isolated. Whether it is to be a standard killed vaccine or one whose virulence has been reduced to allow it to be used as a living vaccine, a long process of adaptation is necessary. To grow well, to be readily harvested and concentrated, means in practice months of testing minor variants of the new virus until one emerges that has all the necessary virtues. If, however, one had a good vaccine strain of A^0 antigenic type available and a totally new strain A^3 against which a vaccine must be made as rapidly as possible, there were real possibilities of finding the right variant much more rapidly. From double infections with A^0 and A^3, one could expect to obtain a wide range of viruses in which the various qualities of the two might be distributed almost at random. With anti-body against A^0 added to the mixture, only viruses with the antigenic (immunizing) quality of A^3 would remain. Amongst them would almost certainly be some with the qualities from A^0 which would make it a good vaccine strain. This was not done in 1957 but a few years later Kilbourne and Murphy showed

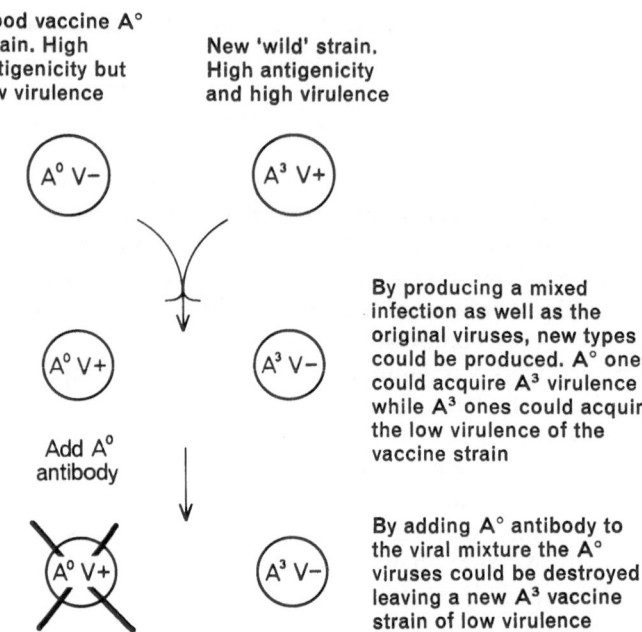

FIG. 22. The production of influenza virus vaccine by recombination.

that it could in fact be done. There will doubtless be other appearances of new influenza viruses in the future and there is always the possibility of exceptionally virulent strains appearing of viruses which we have come to regard as producing only trivial infections. In either eventuality the recombination approach will need to be kept in mind. That calls up the second potentially significant impact of virus genetics on human affairs, the possible production —by accident or deliberately—of unnaturally virulent and dangerous viruses. Outside of science fiction I cannot really picture some omniscient microbiologist inserting a few changed nucleotides into a polio virus and blackmailing the world. But in 1966 I was worried and to a certain extent still am, over the possibility of taking antigen character from one and virulence from another of two currently harmless viruses and combing them to produce something very dangerous. I was thinking particularly of the polio viruses and some of their near relatives.

The three polio viruses, Types I, II, and III, are classified according to the type of immunity they produce. In most respects they are very similar but infection with I immunizes only against itself and the other two are equally individual. A vaccine must therefore be made from all three types. The other significant feature of the polio viruses is that they belong to a much larger group of generally similar viruses found in the intestines of human beings and many other mammals. About sixty-three have been isolated from human material. Each of the sixty-three is antigenically distinct: none will produce effective immunity against any other one. Some of the sixty viruses, other than the three polio types, produce minor human illnesses and one is a very rare producer of polio but in general only the three polio viruses are important. At the present time most human beings, either as a result of immunization or by harmless natural infection, have immunity against the three sorts of polio. In the more crowded areas of the tropics most will have a fairly wide range of immunities to the other sixty intestinal viruses but in the affluent communities of temperate climates there will be few of these immunities.

In any crowded urban environment with poor sanitary facilities the polio viruses spread freely amongst infants and very young children producing as a rule very little evidence of paralysis. These invisible (subclinical) infections immunize the children in very much the same way that a dose of Sabin's living vaccine vaccine does. If, by living in rural isolation or otherwise, a person reaches adult life without ever meeting a polio virus, he is considerably more likely to be paralysed than a young child would be, when he is eventually infected. Towards the end of the Second World War, Malta suffered a severe polio epidemic with numerous cases in young Maltese children, but there were none in Maltese children over the age of 5. On the other hand there were many cases in young English servicemen, especially those brought up in the country. When, in the days before immunization, polio invaded an isolated region, usually an island, where it had been absent for many years the main impact of paralysis was on young adults. This is the characteristic feature of the 'virgin soil' epidemic. One on St. Helena in 1947 is a good example.

It will be clear that what worries me is the possibility that a virulent polio virus might achieve an antigenic character which would be essentially new to the world's population. Nothing could

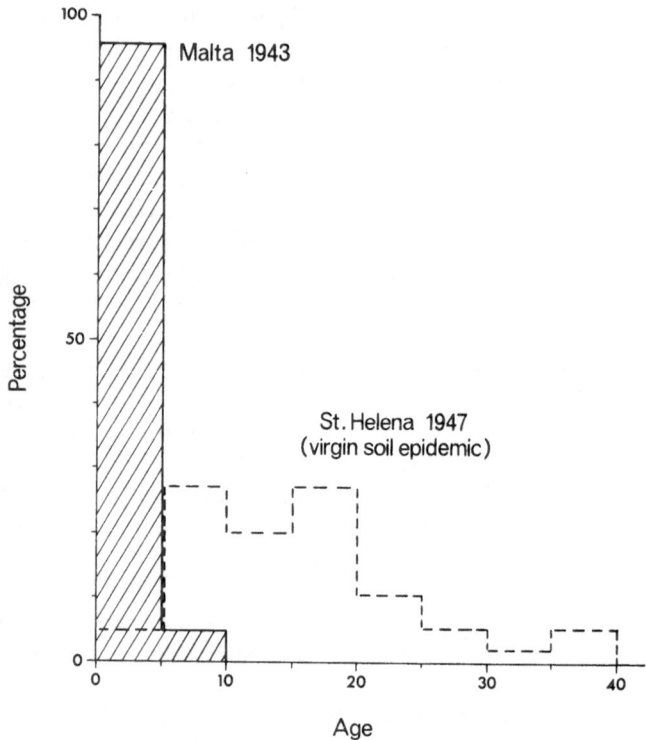

F IG. 23. The percentages of cases in various age-groups in two polio epidemics before the days of immunization (*a*) in a crowded urban community (Malta); (*b*) in an isolated island (St Helena).

be more disastrous than a virgin soil epidemic of polio involving the world or even a single large city. This is very unlikely to occur naturally; we have been watching polio now for over ninety years and if a new antigenic type were going to arise we should have seen it by now. I do not think that this, however, eliminates the possibility of its arising by accident in a laboratory engaged on genetic studies with polio and related viruses. There are potent ways of increasing mutation rates, there are highly selective environments that can be applied and easy ways to cause a given mutant to proliferate to almost any order of magnitude. An additional factor is that human beings working for years with viruses to which they know they are immune are liable to become a little careless.

This long discussion about what must appear very remote contingencies, has two objectives. The first is to underline the possibility that human action can produce biological dangers which could never arise within a natural ecological system. The second is to indicate how far beyond the bounds of the practical it is to look for deliberate chemical rearrangement of the nucleotide units in DNA or RNA to produce a predictable result even with the smallest 'organism' of practical importance.

Transfer of genetic information

We are not, however, necessarily limited to actual chemical manipulations in producing deliberate modification of genetic character.

The DNA of bacteria is at present far too complex to be sorted out chemically but as I have already described, Avery in 1943, was able to induce genetic change in a bacterium, the pneumococcus with DNA from another sort of pneumococcus. Much work has been done on this 'transformation' phenomenon since 1943. Its essential feature can probably be summarized by saying that transformation only occurs in a small proportion of the bacteria exposed to the transforming DNA and that in each case it represents the incorporation of only a small unit of DNA into *the right place* in the DNA repository of the recipient bacterium. There it replaces the original segment and establishes itself as part of the bacterial cell's inheritable mechanism.

A few years later, two other methods of transferring genetic information from one bacterium to another were developed. Quite surprisingly at the time it was found that a strain of *E. coli* and its variants could show what were equivalent to male and female forms. Under appropriate situations the male and female forms would fuse and a string of DNA pass from male (F+) to female (F−), transferring genetic qualities to be expressed in the female cell's progeny. The situation is actually more complex than that, as the capacity for a bacterium to be male (F+ or Hfr) is transmissible as if it were a virus-like agent. The next discovery was that when one uses low virulence bacterial viruses and transfers them from one type of bacterial host *A* to another recognizably different one *B*, a proportion of cultures from infected *B* show some of the characters of *A*. As *A* is being converted into virus particles, fragments of bacterial DNA seem to be trapped in the capsule of the virus and can be conveyed to the DNA of *B* in much the same

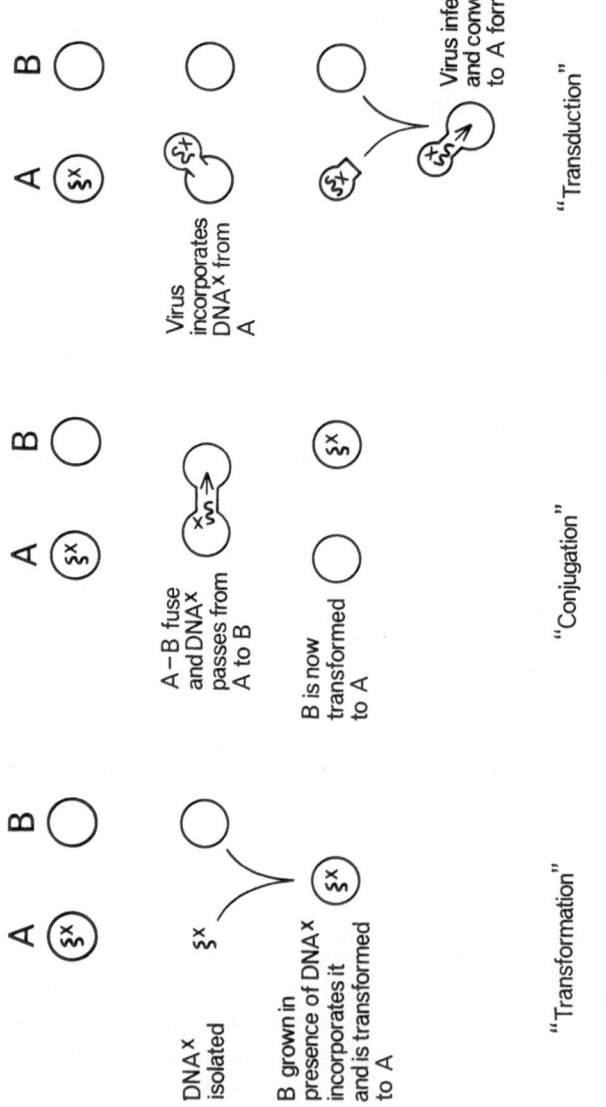

FIG. 24. Three ways in which DNA carrying a particular genetic character can be transferred from one bacterial strain to another so conferring type *A* qualities on type *B*.

way as happens in Avery's experiment. Much more recently, Japanese bacteriologists found disconcertingly that a culture of bacteria that had developed resistance to several antibiotics could transfer that resistance to an initially sensitive bacterium. Such transfers are now referred to as due to R-factors. Their importance is obvious because of the ease with which the changed form will grow in an animal or man under antibiotic treatment.

These genetic changes in bacteria have now been well known for years and they provide much of the background for speculation about what can be done by manipulating genetic material. Much scholarly acclaim has been bestowed on these discoveries but as an ecologically minded scientist I am disappointed that no investigator has made any successful effort to find whether any of these phenomena can be recognized in the natural habitats of bacteria or has tried by indirect approaches to deduce whether they played a part in the evolution of bacteria.

The R factor is important in that man-made ecological niche, the patient treated with antibiotics, but that is a basically artificial situation. I have an uneasy feeling which I fancy that professional bacterial geneticists will scoff at, that in all these phenomena we are exploiting a variety of structural weaknesses in organisms which are too small and primitive to maintain 100 per cent of structural integrity. When the experimenter is handling organisms which proliferate rapidly and where he can devise selective situations where only the type of variant he expects or wants to find can grow, then he is bound to find such variants if they ever arise. All the phenomena are quite probably artifacts in the sense that they play no part in bacterial evolution. Nevertheless, if an artificial situation can be devised and elaborated which throws light on the structure of genetic material in bacteria, this is a completely legitimate scientific approach. Equally, because something has played no part in evolution, there is no reason why it should not be twisted to human benefit or, more often, human ill.

Before any thought is given to the possibilities that in some way these tricks of passing pieces of DNA from one bacterium to another could be applied to human problems, there is one crucially important point to be remembered. There must be a highly selective environment to sort out the mutant hybrid or recombinant. Very often there will be a million unchanged bacteria for the one we want.

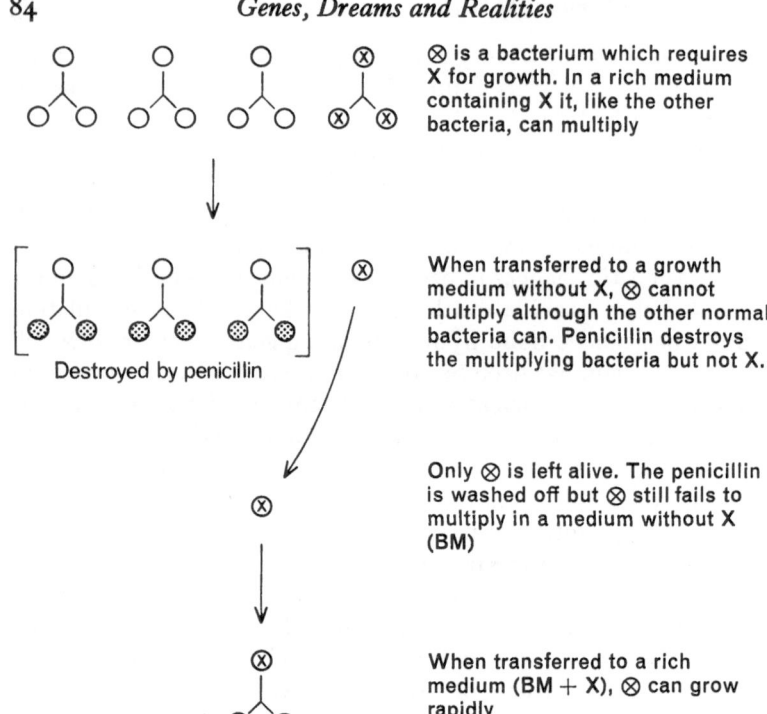

FIG. 25. The use of penicillin to isolate a 'deficient' bacterial mutant.

In Chapter 1, I spoke of isolating a penicillin-resistant mutant by an extremely simple procedure. Suppose, however, we are investigating the chemical reactions of bacteria in the same sort of way that Beadle and Tatum worked with their mould *Neurospora*. Our standard strain of *E. coli* will grow well on a basic medium BM with only a simple sugar, ammonia, and the necessary inorganic ions but it will grow rather better on a rich bacteriological broth with a wide variety of amino acids and other organic molecules available for its nutrition. At various stages of our research we may need a mutant which cannot make some necessary metabolite, amino acid *X* for example, and which can therefore only multiply when *X* is supplied in the growth medium. Here the procedure is more complex, in fact it is so ingenious that it provides a minor intelligence test for any layman who attempts to follow the reasoning! The key to the method is that penicillin can kill only growing bacteria; if, for any reason, they cannot grow, penicillin is quite harmless to them. We start with a culture of *E. coli* which has been growing on a bacteriological broth with all the amino acids available. Some mutants that *need X* are almost certainly present. The problem is to isolate them from the unchanged millions. The procedure, in brief, is to wash away all the rich medium, transfer the bacteria to basal medium with a dose of penicillin lethal for all bacteria that can grow in BM. The next step is again to wash the bacteria (alive and dead) this time to get rid of all penicillin, place a large number of the washed bacteria into two culture bottles, one BM, the other BM+X, and incubate them for some hours. If all has gone well, there will be no growth in BM but in BM+X there will be a turbidity to show where the wanted mutant is growing. The one-in-a-million that was needed has been isolated.

Genetically a man and a bacterium are each individuals. The likelihood of slipping some desirable genetic quality into the next human generation is in any sense utterly remote but suppose it were decided to try by treating spermatozoa with DNA extract from some esoteric source. If 100 million sperms are treated, one would, on bacterial analogies, produce a hundred or two hundred insertions of the new DNA of which probably 90 per cent would not 'work properly'. The problem becomes, to find the dozen or so 'good' sperm in 100 million. I need not elaborate the difficulty.

It will be more convenient to defer any detailed discussion of what would be needed to handle a case of genetic disease along such lines until these diseases are dealt with in Chapter 6. But we can return briefly to the two suggestions for genetic engineering which I drew from Kornberg and Tatum at the beginning of this chapter to emphasize their impracticability and dangers. In the Kornberg approach the synthetic gene is implanted in one of the 'cancer viruses' and ferried to all the relevant cells of the patient by injection of large amounts of treated virus into the blood circulation. Tatum's suggestion was to treat a tissue culture of the patient's cells with the 'good' gene, sort out the tiny proportion that would be 'cured' and grow them up to the required bulk for implantation into the patient. My objections to both are: *first*, it is highly improbable that the necessary experiments could ever be done to find the right conditions needed to benefit the *individual* human patient that we must always have in mind. Men are all genetically unique; they are not pure line mice; *second*, it is inevitable that the injection of such material into the patient irrespective of how far the difficulties of producing it have been overcome, would be as likely to induce malignant disease as to provide new genetic capacity to the patient. Neither approach has yet been tried and I doubt whether they ever *will* be tried by responsible investigators.

CELLULAR MANIPULATION

Replacement of faulty clones of cells

The only claim that I am aware of to have righted a genetic deficiency involved the different principle of actually transplanting a cell population congenitally absent or ineffective and doing what seemed necessary to prevent rejection of the transplant by the child's immune response. The patient was a child with a congenitally undeveloped thymus and all the immune deficiencies that go with such a condition. Sooner or later it would be lethal. One thing that happens in such children is for their vaccination against smallpox to fail to heal completely and to kill the child with spreading ulceration at the site and generalization to the rest of the body. The child in question was treated by transplanting a graft of bone marrow from his sister on the assumption that the thymus had failed to develop because it was not being supplied with stem cells of the right type from the bone marrow. Since the patient had no immune capacity to reject a foreign graft, his sister's bone marrow cells established themselves selectively and within a week or two it was clear that the child's thymus and immune system were functioning. Then complications set in and the child developed a rapid and severe anaemia. The patient's new immune system was *someone else's* to which the patient's red cells and many other cells were foreign. It could not therefore avoid mounting an attack on those of the host's bone marrow cells which were functioning, hence the anaemia.

The all-wise haematologist was at hand, however, and at the right moment a second bone marrow transplantation from the sister resulted in a complete restocking of blood cells, red and white, stem cells in the bone marrow and defence cells, all from the sister. Now it appears that the boy will live happily ever after—although not all immunologists are as optimistic as the team who reported the case. It may well be that the time is not yet ripe—the Hippocratic oath, religious teaching, and the opinions that people express in public all stand in the way—but some of us would quite seriously advise that such children, lacking inherited capacity for normal immunity, should be given no more than simple treatment for their inevitable infections. Here, at least, negative euthanasia is the only humanitarian approach.

Biological cryogenics

Before closing this chapter on the 'exciting new' approaches to curing disease or changing the quality of human life, a little should be said about the alleged possibilities of prolonging life indefinitely by freezing the whole individual. In the previous chapter I said something about the application of intense cold to the preservation of bull spermatozoa in a viable state. This is the only really practical application yet of biological cryogenics but it is a sub-science with many uses in the laboratory. If cells can be so preserved it is natural to ask whether with adequately painstaking research, it should not be possible to freeze the body so that viability was retained indefinitely. Obviously, both the freezing and thawing processes would be critical but if the requirements were only technical, no doubt appropriate techniques could be developed.

In science fiction such a method is thought of as the only way by which a space-ship could reach a relatively near solar system with living human beings aboard. They would, of course, have to be thawed by a computer programmed some centuries earlier! There are, however, claims for the potentialities of such methods nearer to home. There are already a few cadavers frozen hard in containers packed with dry ice or liquid nitrogen. They are waiting, we are told, in the expectation that the swift advance of medical science will in due course make it possible (*a*) to bring back to life a person who had died *x* years previously, provided he had been held at the proper temperature, and (*b*) to cure the condition from which he had died. It would be logical to add a third future achievement of medicine as (*c*) to produce the Faustian miracle of reversing the changes of age and endowing perpetual youthful maturity on the resurrected.

Every well-informed biologist knows that there has never been a successful recovery after freezing solid a vertebrate animal, and most are convinced that the physical and chemical difficulties will always be too great to allow successful return to life. On the other hand it is well known that appropriate handling to avoid the development of ice crystals in cell substance will allow the indefinite storage at the temperature of liquid nitrogen of a variety of mammalian cells including spermatozoa of some species, notably of cattle. This is enough to allow optimistically minded physiologists to feel that prolonged experiments on animals might eventually lead to a highly sophisticated technique by which the various difficulties of the blood circulation could be dealt with. To avoid damage to the highly susceptible cells of the brain and spinal cord would be still more difficult and, as yet, there is no suggestion as to how they could be turned off to remain viable indefinitely, and in due course be turned on again in full function. I do not expect it to happen but I would not quite dare to predict that a century of intensive research would still be fruitless. What can be said very firmly, however, is that until a research team can in 99 per cent of cases freeze a dog for three months and on 'resurrecting' it show that it still possesses the memory and intelligence it showed previously, it would be utter charlatanry to advocate the sort of thing we are now hearing about from America.

Should those dogs eventually pass all their tests, then it is just conceivable that in the distant future some healthy young men and women may volunteer to be subjected to the same procedure with the promise of special privilege and prestige when they are revived one hundred years later. That, of course, is straightforward science fiction but it would still be far away from the requirements (*a*), (*b*), and (*c*) of today's 'resurrection men'. Death, if it has any biological meaning in these days of organ transplantation, iron lungs, artificial kidneys, and heart-lung machines, represents the irreversible disorganization of nerve cell function in the brain, in most cases due to a few minutes' lack of oxygen through failure of the circulation. Once that has occurred there is no faintest possibility in sight of reorganizing it—'All the king's horses and all the king's men couldn't put Humpty together again.' This being the case, it is quite useless and tedious to run through the various reasons why terminal cancer would remain incurable, and the cellular changes of old age remain irreversible, even if the corpse could in some sense be brought back to life.

I have heard one enthusiast on a television programme speak of the preservation of the dead for scientific resurrection as the great trillion-dollar industry of the future. It is a statement that may throw some light on the social psychoses of our time but it is not one for the investing public to take seriously—nor for the demographers to look at as a new nightmare to plague them.

5

THE TWO CATEGORIES: EXTERNAL
IMPACT AND INTERNAL EXPRESSION

I have already indicated how disease and disability can be divided
into two categories with only a minor residue that remains indeter-
minate. There are first those conditions which result from the
impact of the environment on individuals who come within the
bounds of the genetically normal. There are, on the other hand,
diseases which spring from processes intrinsic to the individual.
They will inevitably be influenced by environmental factors but
such factors will be ineffective in most other individuals. The
great successes of medicine are to be found in the first group. In
the second, we are concerned amongst other things with old age,
cancer, and natural death.

THE POSITIVE ACHIEVEMENTS OF MEDICAL SCIENCE

The great successes of medicine have been concerned with what
comes from without—infection, nutrition, injury. Conditions due
to these impacts of the environment are nowadays usually easy to
recognize though they may not have been so in the past. Where it
is difficult to be sure about a given instance it is almost always
because genetic and other intrinsic factors are unusually significant.
In the group of infections, one includes general and localized
infections by micro-organisms—measles and a boil on the neck
can serve as examples—and we must bring into the net larger
organisms from the amoeba of dysentery to hydatid cysts of the
liver.

Under nutritional inadequacies there is a large range, from
starvation and acute protein deficiency in children (kwashiorkor)
to specific vitamin or mineral deficiencies—and one must include
a variety of acute or chronic poisonings.

Injury by misadventure, criminal action, or war, can take a
thousand forms: wounding, burning, drowning, and the rest.

G.D.R.—7

It is merely to state the obvious that in a community with advanced medical care, all these things can be effectively dealt with. Anyone with an interest in what happens in the world will have some appreciation of such landmarks in the development of that success as sulpha drugs, blood transfusion, the anti-rickets vitamin D, penicillin, and DDT. The task of dealing medically with the impact of the environment is now in principle virtually complete; in practice there will always be scope for improvement. In our particular context and in 1971, the most important need is to realize why it was relatively easy to deal with all the problems from the environment. In due course this will throw light on the difficulties of handling the intrinsic problems.

When we try to look for the basic reasons for success, they seem to be three:

1. Anything from the environment that is harmful to a man or a child is likely to be harmful in somewhat similar fashion to mouse or rabbit or monkey. It may be hard to find the right species of animal or arrange the right conditions but eventually a good animal model of the disease or disability has almost always been produced. Once that is available the condition is subject to controlled investigation for ways of preventing or curing it.

No condition induced in a laboratory animal will be a complete model of a human illness and unrealized differences have often delayed a proper understanding of some human disease. Every model needs to be critically considered in the light of the human problem. sometimes rather unnatural models must be used. Leprosy has been notoriously difficult to produce in animals but recently inoculation of leprosy tissue into the feet of mice whose immune system had been paralysed by removal of the thymus gland has given something very like lepromatous leprosy. It may well turn out to be an excellent model on which to assess drugs for the treatment of lepromatous leprosy in man.

Examples could be given in every field. The great life-saving discoveries, the ones for which Nobel prizes were won, almost all came from the interaction between laboratory experiment on animals and careful clinical trial.

2. These environmental causes of illness are nearly all conditions which, once looked at carefully, can be understood at the level of ordinary human experience. A hundred years ago the notion of

invisible microbes causing infectious disease may have been difficult to grasp, but to most people it is nowadays accepted as simple common sense.

What one eats has always been regarded as significant for health and the ideas of vitamins or of bacteriological control of food and water were readily grasped and acted upon. All these things look like straightforward examples of cause and effect. This is emphasized simply to point up the extreme difficulty that many people have in understanding the quite different sort of logic which must be applied to many of the intrinsic conditions.

3. The third reason for satisfaction is the *effectiveness* with which, when social and economic conditions are right, these things can be dealt with. The current methods of immunization against diphtheria and poliomyelitis have virtually eliminated both diseases from Western countries. A hundred years ago the mortality was frighteningly high for persons with severe pneumonia, men suffering from starvation and exposure, or soldiers with gunshot wounds. Today we feel confident that nearly all such victims can look forward to recovery and effectively complete rehabilitation if only they can reach modern medical care before the damage done has become irreversibly lethal. There will always be a minority of failures, and an interesting aspect of modern medicine has emerged as a result. When a cure that works with almost every case of condition X fails, it is very likely that what looked like X was really Y. Quite a number of 'new' diseases have been detected as a result. Pneumonia, for example, became an eminently curable disease when the second generation of sulpha drugs appeared and even more so with the advent of penicillin. A pneumonia in a young person which could not be cured in a day or two, obviously was not real *Pneumococcus* pneumonia. It had to have another name and quickly became 'Atypical pneumonia' which in due course was shown to result from infection by a totally different micro-organism (*Mycoplasma*).

There is a fourth consideration that may be relevant in a somewhat different way. Only a professional biologist would ever be likely to raise it—the social usefulness of the man or woman who has recovered from serious illness. In nature, chronic illness cannot exist; a sick animal dies soon under the attack of predators or from starvation. Without pressing the analogy, a healthy person is an asset to the state, a chronically disabled one a liability. Nearly always the social usefulness of an individual is far more likely to be conserved following effective treatment of externally originating disability than after any of the more serious intrinsic conditions. This may have important implications for medical care policy in developing countries.

In principle all the environmentally arising disabilities were understood and could be effectively treated or prevented by 1955. If it were socially and economically practical to apply world-wide the best level of medical and surgical practice that was available in 1955, 99 per cent of people would be receiving better, for the most part infinitely better, medical care than they can actually obtain in 1971. Of course there have been improvements since 1955 in ways of handling trauma and infection and there will always be opportunity for the intelligent, enthusiastic group with some special interest to improve results beyond those achieved by the average competent practitioner or hospital. When it comes, however, to looking for improvements in principle needed for the future, there is not a great deal to be seen in prospect. It is probably characteristic of the time that little about improving these fields of medicine appears in the popular Press or on television programmes.

Looked at from a technical angle the important problems at the present time seem to be the following.:

1. The provision of improved antibiotics, antimalarials, and medically significant insecticides to deal with organisms that have developed intrinsic resistance. This is part of the inevitable result of interference with ecological systems; it will probably always be unavoidable and technical developments have so far kept pace with requirements.

2. An understanding of the viruses concerned with infectious hepatitis (jaundice) and the serum hepatitis that may follow blood transfusion. The discovery of the so-called Australia antigen three years ago makes it likely that practical solutions to both problems can be looked for. Progress so far has been slow.

3. In the underprivileged world there are many sources of infection or worm infestation which cannot be dealt with by means that are effective in affluent societies. These call for cheaper approaches. The most important is for ways to deal with schistosomiasis, the

worm infestation of bowel and bladder which ranges through most of Africa. Water snails are the important intermediary and the current approach is to develop molluscicides to deal with snails without serious upset to other ecological factors. The eye disease trachoma probably comes next in importance and malaria is still very far from being eliminated.

Perhaps one could sum up the position in regard to medical control of the impact of the environment by saying that from the demographic, social, and economic angle this is the only aspect of modern medicine that has mattered. The population explosion derives from its success, the health of the work force depends upon it and military medicine is concerned with nothing else.

INTRINSIC SOURCES OF DISEASE

If we set aside the impact of the environment, scientific medicine is concerned essentially with preventing or delaying death that seems likely to result from genetic anomalies, germinal or somatic, presented by the individual. This is a harshly limited statement which leaves uncovered the largest area of any general practitioner or physician's professional work. For the purpose of this book I am virtually forgetting the personal relationship of doctor and patient, the anxieties, fears, and hopes of sick people and the social responsibilities of the doctor as he sees them against the traditional culture and ethics of his community. Also excluded is the wide range of conditions which rank as diseases and are ascribed to mental and emotional causes, as psychosomatic, psychoneurotic, or hysterical conditions. Such an exclusion is only justifiable for the specific reason that the book, as such, is primarily aimed at clarifying the part played by genetic factors in disease and in trying to forecast future developments in that field.

The genetic diseases proper are important but not nearly so important in my view as those that are the result of deviations in somatic genetics. I believe that a discussion of the possibilities of dealing with the commoner genetic diseases can be given in Chapter 6 without any preliminary words here. My experience in teaching on somatic genetics, however, leaves me convinced that this does require as clear a presentation as I can provide of general principles before specific discussion of ageing and cancer.

In Chapter 1, I spoke about the necessity of looking at conditions

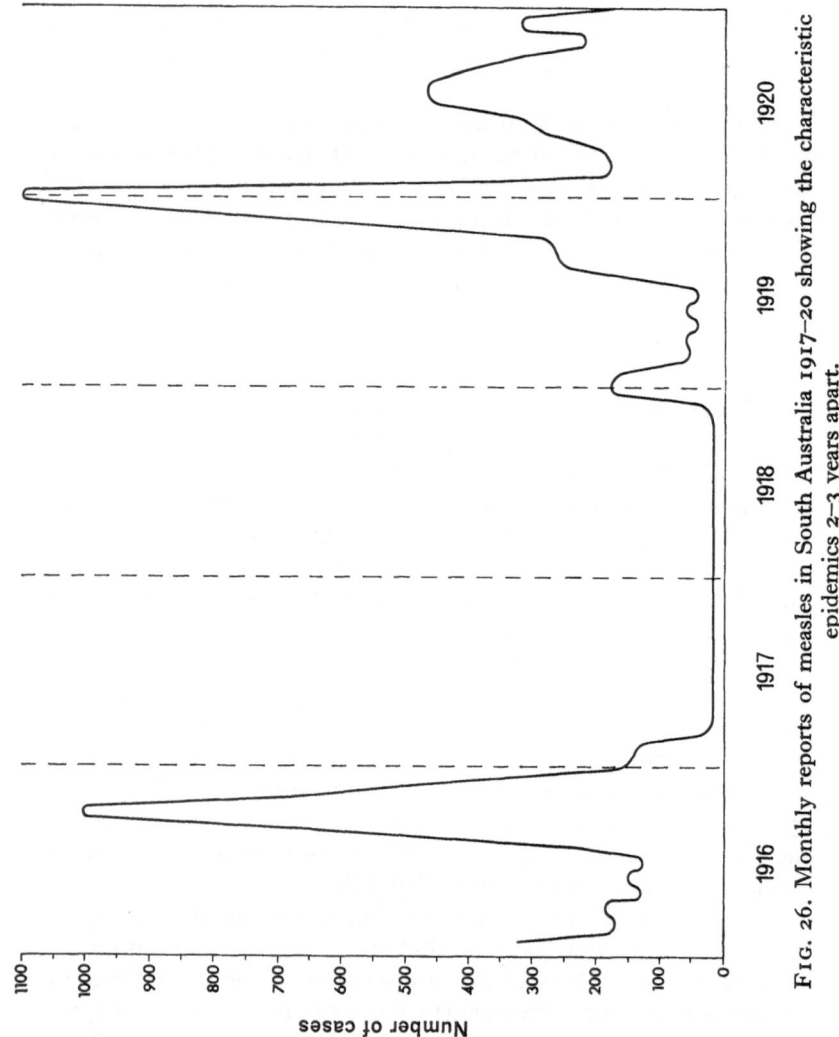

Fig. 26. Monthly reports of measles in South Australia 1917–20 showing the characteristic epidemics 2–3 years apart.

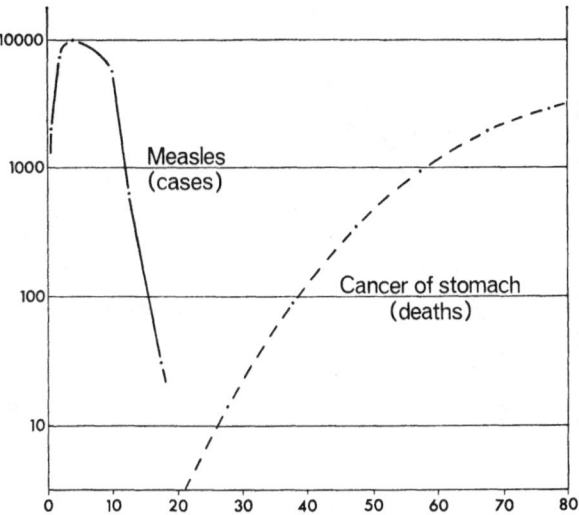

FIG. 27. A graph contrasting the age incidence of measles and gastric cancer.

that were or might be based on random processes such as somatic mutation from a stochastic rather than a determinative point of view. At the risk of some repetition, one can say that the essence of the stochastic approach to any type of disease is to realize that the occurrence of that disease in any particular individual was wholly unpredictable. The occurrence only becomes susceptible to scientific study as a statistic.

Any disease that can be defined and diagnosed will attract the interest of statisticians and epidemiologists. There will be on record somewhere for every individual who died of disease X, whether it was typhoid fever, cancer of the stomach, or road accident, a group of basic facts. There will be the patient's sex and age, the date of his death and possibly of the onset of his illness, and the city or district where death occurred. For most infectious diseases there are similar data in regard to both fatal and non-fatal cases and there are many other non-lethal conditions like shingles (*herpes zoster*), Bell's palsy (facial paralysis), or Graves's disease (toxic goitre), which have been studied sufficiently widely to give the same information about who, when, and where.

When one has records of a thousand or more cases of disease

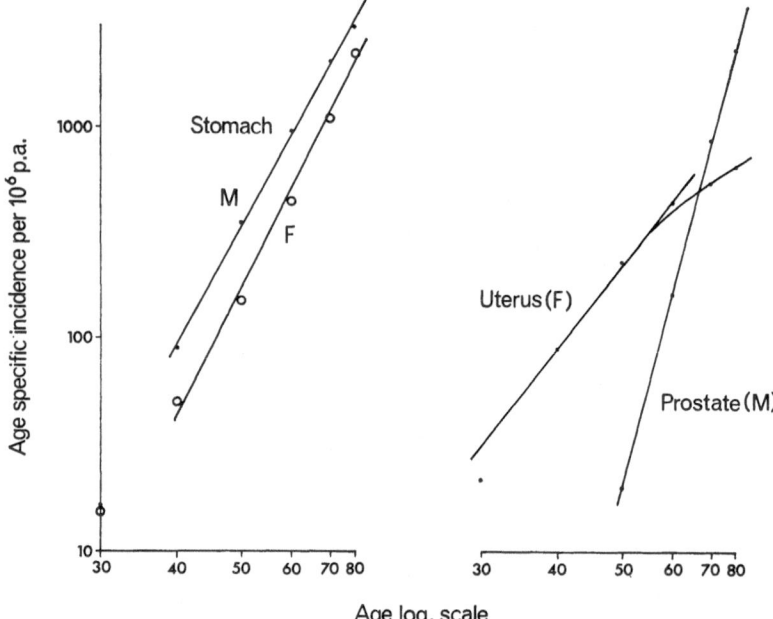

F I G. 28. Graphs showing stochastic regularities in four types of cancer. All are age-specific incidence of death plotted log./log. from England and Wales figures 1950–4.

1 and 2 Stomach cancer male and female showing close approximation to two parallel straight lines.
3   Uterus showing how incidence rises less rapidly in old age.
4   Prostate showing the abnormally steep incidence in old age.

from a city or from a reasonably homogeneous country, tables can be made and graphs can be drawn. Reported cases of measles and deaths from cancer of the stomach may be taken. We want to avoid getting caught in the complexities that come into any actual figures so I shall only show the simplified essence of the contrasting curves.

The first curves show the dates at which each case or death was recorded over a period of five years. Then we have the 'age-specific incidence' which is the percentage of cases in each particular five-year age-group relative to the total number of persons in each such age-group. In measles epidemics every mother knows that any children who have not already had measles and are going to school will catch it. She also knows that once a child has had measles he is immune for life. With those simple rules and common sense any intelligent layman could see the age-specific incidence curve for measles is what he would expect. That for gastric cancer is just about as different as it can possibly be. In the first place, 95 per cent of people get recognized measles, while only 1 or 2 per cent of people die of stomach cancer. Cancer always seems to be a disease of the old but it is better expressed as a disease which becomes increasingly more likely with each year after about the age of 40.

This somewhat self-evident discussion is simply to demonstrate the way in which disease incidence can be represented. The specific age incidence curve is the most significant and can in fact provide much information. Anywhere in the world the curve for gastric cancer would take that general form but in detail there would be interesting differences. It would rise nearly three times as high in Japan as in Europe, for example, and there is much investigation going on in Japan to trace a reason for the difference. Curves of this type can be studied mathematically as representing stochastic processes where things happen at random for the individual but according to regular laws for a large enough population.

On a much broader scale it is perfectly legitimate to say that the whole evolution of life has been based on random errors which on a large enough scale over a long enough time have, as it were, constructed their own laws for evolutionary progress. Evolution emerges from three sets of stochastic (random, yet subject to law) processes—mutation within the germ line, recombination by sexual reproduction of genetic patterns and selective survival of populations.

In this chapter we are only very remotely concerned with evolution in the ordinary sense but, if we are interested in ageing and the diseases of age including cancer, then a pseudo-evolutionary approach to differentiation, somatic mutation, and selective survival amongst the cells of the body becomes positively mandatory. No reasonable predictions about future applications of biology to medicine can be made unless the full implications of this approach are understood. Medical science must always work with individuals who are born and die, and every general practitioner of medicine will inevitably be concerned now and for as long as there are doctors and patients, very largely with those 'on the wrong side of 50'. Before discussing prospects of changing approaches to old age and cancer in Chapters 7 and 8, I want to do my best to clarify the necessary approach. A broad outline was given in the introductory chapter. Here we must exemplify some of the cellular changes at the level both of individual cells and of cell populations that lead to 'intrinsic' disease.

The body as a population of cells

The cells of the body differ almost as much in appearance and function as at a higher level the different species of mammal differ one from another. All cells have a dynamic history during the progressive stages of differentiation and growth, but differences begin to be evident very early. In a grown man or any other mammal some cells have ended their growth for ever, some can only multiply for emergency reasons while others will continue proliferating until, and perhaps even a little after, death.

When we are looking at the body as essentially a population of cells it is advisable first to grasp what portion of the body structure is made up of non-cellular material and to have some idea of how this is related to the living cellular components. The second aspect which is intensely relevant is what we can call the population dynamics, the manifest destiny, or the natural history—call it what you will—of the various cells within the body. This applies specially to those cell types which are continually multiplying but in many ways almost equally to those which only proliferate to help repair damage or are permanently non-multiplying so that the only possible population change is diminution by death. These aspects can be expounded under five headings, two concerned with the non-cellular components of the body, three with the cell types I have mentioned.

1. The solid non-cellular components are essentially crystalline minerals and protein fibres in molecular form. The former are limited to bone and teeth: the fibres are universal. If it became possible to remove miraculously all cells from the body, as well as all free fluid, one would have something that was still the shape of a man and probably still as difficult to disintegrate. The bones would probably seem little changed, there would be dense fibrous bundles in all tendons, capsules, and the like, and through every functional organ, shape, and structure would be broadly recognizable by fine

networks of fibres. The bones are to a large extent calcium salts (apatite) crystallized on a framework of collagen fibres. These fibres and another type (elastin) provide structure and toughness for all parts of the body and are correspondingly close-packed where toughness is most needed. The fibres are not living; they are bundles of rather simply constructed protein molecules, linked chains of amino acids, which can be as long or as short as the body needs. They are just molecules but they are intimately related to the cells which produce them and the equally important but little understood cells which remove damaged or unnecessary fibres. Collagen and elastin being as important for effective function as any system of cells, we know that every group of fibres has been laid down and moulded by processes developed during evolution to do the job properly. There are good indications that mechanical tension will ensure maintenance and, if necessary, strengthening of the local collagen bundles but in general we cannot do much more than accept that collagen and elastin are *there* in position and amount appropriate to function.

2. The blood and lymph fluids are non-living but immensely complex, probably containing molecules of every soluble substance in the body. The blood plasma is subject to perpetual dynamic change and it is a fair summary to say that every one of the components which has been found to be of physiological importance is subject to a balanced (homeostatic) control. The complexity and control reach such a degree that if a physologist should proclaim that the whole of the blood fluid was *really* a formless and dilute kind of living substance, I might disagree but I know that the argument would only be a semantic one.

3. The first group of cells to be noted are those which once they have been laid down can never be replaced. The nerve cells of brain and spinal cord are the outstanding examples since they are incapable of proliferation or of repair when their axons—the threads of protoplasm that remotely resemble the lines in a telephone system or the wiring of a computer—are severed. Fish and frog can carry out such repairs but not mammals. In man and laboratory mammals peripheral nervous tissue can regenerate severed axons and traumatized or denervated muscle can be brought back to function by cellular repair and hypertrophy but neither

type can multiply. It is significant that tumours of nerve cells or voluntary muscle cells are extraordinarily rare.

4. For a number of reasons the capacity of liver cells to regenerate and multiply has been deeply studied. In the normal liver, one finds only a very small proportion of the liver cells proper showing any sign of division. But if a substantial fraction of the liver is removed surgically or a similar proportion of the cells killed by an appropriate dose of carbon tetrachloride, the surviving cells rapidly begin to proliferate. Essentially similar results are seen when portion of the kidney is removed. In both organs the proliferation of cells provides a basis for the reconstruction of new regions of functioning tissue. Similar limitation of cell proliferation to the repair of injury can be seen in a number of other organs.

5. When we are considering body cells as dynamic populations we are naturally chiefly concerned with those types which multiply freely. It is equally obvious that since the adult body remains in dynamic equilibrium we must be as much concerned with the concomitant destruction of cells which maintains the balance. For our present purposes it is a legitimate simplification to reduce such cells to two groups, circulating cells and the epithelial cells covering external and internal surfaces. In both groups there can usually be recognized a population of 'stem cells', i.e., cells of fairly primitive unspecialized character which for the most part multiply quietly producing descendants exactly like themselves in number sufficient to maintain their numbers. Under appropriate demand for differentiated descendants some individual stem cells commence to multiply more actively and as they do so, progressively differentiate into specialized cells.

The typical epithelial layers are the skin and the cells that line the stomach and intestines or the air passages. In all there is a constant wearing away of superficial cells and their balanced replacement from the stem cell reservoir. In the skin the stem cells form a basal layer from which new cells proliferate and as they move upward become progressively horny and are eventually lost as dry flakes of keratin. There are different, but essentially equivalent, arrangements to replenish the cells lost from internal linings.

From many points of view the stem cells in the bone marrow are the most important of all. With the proviso that it is technically extraordinarily difficult to trace origins and migrations of cells

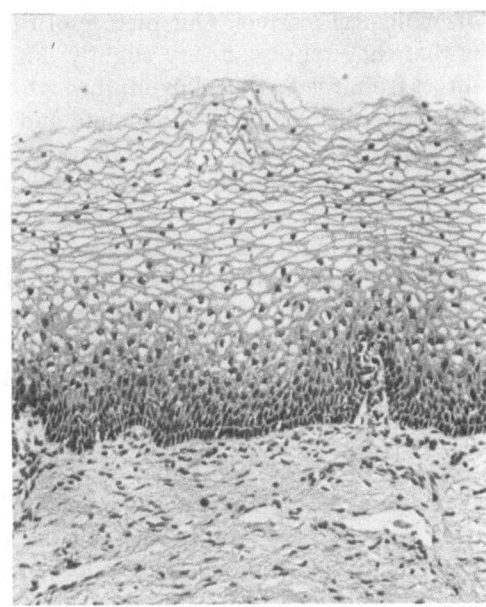

FIG. 29. A skin section showing cells from which there is constant replacement of cells shed from the surface.

within the body, it is consistent with the known facts to trace all the circulating and mobile cells to the bone marrow.

Amongst the cells in this group are all the blood cells—the red blood cells that carry haemoglobin, all the white cells or leucocytes, including the phagocytes that become evident as pus cells when they have to deal with a serious bacterial invasion, the larger phagocytic monocytes and the versatile lymphocytes which subserve many defensive processes. White cells of all these types can be found in the tissues and it is at least highly probable that the various wandering or settled cells not concerned with the primary function of the tissue, lymphocytes, fibroblasts, macrophages, are derived from the same stem cells.

It is as well to state firmly here that it is quite impossible in principle or in practice to pick a bone marrow cell of undifferentiated appearance and say what are its potentialities. It could be a completely differentiated lymphocyte or it could have potentiality to give rise to any of the circulating or tissue cells I have mentioned.

If one is to avoid being impossibly equivocal, one must pick what seems to be the best general interpretation which has not yet been proved wrong. This holds for almost every general statement on biological matters. Our picture of the bone marrow stem cells is that they represent very slightly differentiated cells that come direct from the fertilized ovum through a line of essentially primitive unspecialized cells. Their fate and that of their descendants depends on their response to local and general hormonal and cell contact stimulation. To offer a trivial human analogy, one can picture 1,000 youths leaving school all of basically normal ability. They will find through employment agencies, Army recruiting depots, family influence, and the rest, a first job. From that, circumstances, ability, and random chance will progressively diversify the population. Amongst the cells we are much more concerned with the combination of proliferation and differentiation which gives rise to the *populations* of cells with which we are essentially concerned.

Deviations from homeostasis

If this book has a persisting theme it is that medical science must now concern itself with ageing and the associated anatomical and functional degenerations, with cancer in all its forms including the conditions we call auto-immune disease—and with the immune responses to such changes which can have both beneficial and harmful results. All these things are based on changes in the populations of cells within the body. A cancer is a malignant uncontrolled proliferation of one type of cell; any infection provokes controlled proliferation of a variety of defence cells and their strategic dispersal through the body. There are cyclical sequences of proliferation and degeneration of cells in breast and uterus which can on occasion break from control. It is at least an expedient and sometimes stimulating approach to subsume such changes under the heading of the population dynamics of body cells with its deliberate implication of a cellular ecology that can on occasion fluctuate beyond normal bounds.

In the final section of this chapter I am only concerned with the processes which will need to be called upon if we are to interpret the important clinical conditions of the intrinsic group. We can accept, without attempting an explanation, the process by which the body reaches and maintains its individual qualities of form and function as *the* fact of life. Since Claude Bernard, the central proposition of mammalian physiology has been the capacity of the body to maintain an approximately constant *milieu interne*. Homeostasis is the first law of mammalian life. It has been studied particularly in regard to the maintenance of the quality of the circulating blood, its temperature, its balance between acidity and alkalinity (pH), the oxygen carried in the red cells. Others have found much the same rules maintained by similar feedbacks and the like for holding the numbers of circulating cells constant except for the changes needed to deal with emergency. Disease may be associated either with undue proliferation of cells or with failure to maintain a particular cell population at a high enough level to allow normal function. At this stage it is sufficient to touch on these only briefly and dogmatically.

Proliferation of cells beyond standard equilibrium levels may be due to:

1. Local or general hormonal stimulation, many of the hormones still being chemically unidentified.

2. Cells of the immune systems carry receptors which are capable of reacting only with the corresponding foreign pattern (antigen). Depending on circumstances, contact with the 'right' antigen will cause the cells to proliferate or cause damage to them which may reach a lethal level.

3. Mutational changes in the cell may render it unresponsive to one or more of the normal controls which maintain structural integrity in the body. This must be postulated for all malignant and benign tumours but there are some important tumours which in addition can only flourish when they are under some particular form of hormonal stimulation.

Failure to maintain standard populations may be due to:

1. The workings of the Hayflick limit—human cells in tissue culture initiated from embryonic cells will go on proliferating under what appear to be optimal conditions, only for about fifty cell generations. It is regarded as likely by Hayflick and others, that this or a similar limit holds for the number of generations a cell line in the body can continue. Others, while accepting the findings in tissue culture, rightly point out that the only reason for considering that a limit exists in the body is to provide some support for speculative theories on the nature of ageing.

2. A variety of destructive actions of immunological character. When one cell reacts immunologically with another cell, one or

both may suffer damage or lethal change. Appropriate antibody may also be lethal to cells but in the body this is probably very rare.

3. The process of cell differentiation and organ building in the embryo involves at many points cell destruction as well as cell proliferation. Everyone is aware of how the tadpole's tail must wither away if the frog is to take its form, and lesser processes of the same general quality are frequent. Some degenerations and disappearances of cells may have to be accepted as a simple manifestation of genetic programming and, as such, no more and no less explicable in detail than the process of development itself.

6

GENETIC DISEASE
THE NATURE OF DIFFERENCES
AMONG MEN

Over the last few years there has been a bitter academic controversy in America on the significance of the fact, admitted by all,
that coloured children have a much lower average IQ than white,
and at the lower level (IQ less than 70) there are 16 per cent of
coloured compared with less than 2 per cent amongst white children. It is equally accepted that the upper limit of IQ is equivalent
to that of whites although there are many fewer coloureds in the
over-130 IQ bracket. The controversy turns on whether most of
these differences depend on upbringing in a disadvantaged community, poor education, and lack of opportunity in the coloured
population or mainly on genetic factors. The official approach, of
the US Office of Education, for instance, is that 'the talent pool
of any one ethnic group is substantially the same as in any other
ethnic group'. This is the view of most academic psychologists and
educationalists and, indeed, it seems to be accepted as at least not
yet disproved and politically expedient to believe by the vast
majority of academics, including the senior scientists of the
National Academy of Science.

This puts the minority who have publicly espoused the genetic
origin of race differences in the role of heretics and the controversy has almost the quality of a religious squabble. The leading
academic on the unpopular side is A. R. Jensen (Professor of
Educational Psychology at Berkeley) whose approach seems to me
an eminently rational one. If the differences are wholly environmental they should be remediable by action against poverty and
compensatory educational privileges. If they are genetic and if
there is, as superficially appears to be the case, a correlation of
genetically low intelligence with location in urban slums, exceptionally high birth-rate, and all the antisocial attributes of such

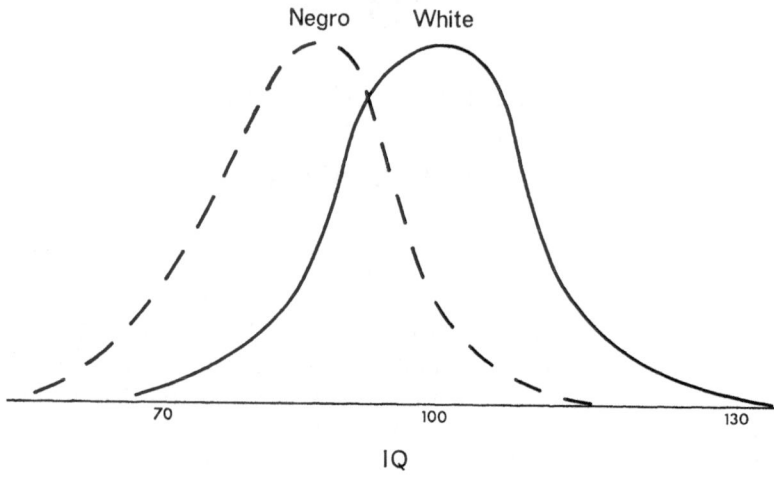

Fɪɢ. 30. The distribution of IQs in whites and Negroes in the United States of America (*Scientific American*, 1970).

populations, then the problem is insoluble except in so far as the eugenic policies can be effectively applied. The claim that a decision is needed as to the relative significance of environmental and genetic factors in determining the distribution of disabling characteristics amongst American Negroes if any rational social policy is to be planned, seems unquestionably correct. Whether in the current temper of American race relations it would be practicable to devise and carry out an adequate scientifically acceptable study, may be another matter.

In all probability the 'heritability' of IQ within negroid or other races, will be close to the 80 per cent found in white populations in Europe and North America, but the extreme genetic heterogeneity of human individuals within any racial group and the impossibility of assessing the influence of all the environmental factors that have played on the individual since his conception could well make it impossible to demonstrate this to any academic emotionally involved on the opposite side.

This introduction to the discussion of genetic disease is there primarily to underline the social and scientific difficulties of dealing with human characteristics which show polygenic inheritance and which are extensively modifiable by environment. These include stature and body configuration, skin colour and probably every character exemplified in behavioural achievement, intelligence, athletic ability, criminality, and the rest. Clear quantitative population genetics requires the study of a few characteristics whose differences depend on one or a very small number of genes. Eye colour, the various blood groups, and a variety of polymorphisms in the structure of blood proteins and enzymes are the ones that have mainly attracted investigators. In every such field, as soon as the numbers of investigated becomes large, exceptions to the regular pattern emerge and have to be accounted for by some abnormal process involving the gene, point-mutation, intragenomic anomalies, or some abnormality of meiosis or fertilization. It can be taken as equally certain that in each of the regions of the genome that control polygenic qualities there is at least the same multiplicity of possible gene reassortments and of new mutation and minor genetic anomaly. One has only to look at the siblings of any reasonably large family of one's acquaintance to see the diversity that can emerge by the reshuffling of the same gene pairs. I believe that for all the qualities that are not clearly and wholly cultural in origin it would be a good working hypothesis to say that the genetic component accounts for 80 per cent of the variance as it has been shown to do in relation to IQ. This almost certainly holds for many of those variations from the norm which constitute or predispose to what we conventionally call disease. One thinks of high blood pressure, susceptibility to arthritis or to tuberculosis, schizophrenia, and schizoid personality. Family studies, comparison of identical twin pairs and non-identical pairs for concordance show that there is some genetic component in them all but there is, as always, an environmental component, which may be as precise and necessary as the tubercle bacillus is in clinical tuberculosis, or very difficult to define as for example in high blood pressure.

Even when we are concerned with abnormalities present at birth we cannot forget the intra-uterine environment in which the foetus has developed. There is a large genetic component in the occurrence of gross anatomical abnormalities like harelip and cleft palate, spina bifida (a failure of the lower part of the spinal cord to develop completely), or pyloric stenosis (an obstructive thickening where the stomach opens into the first part of the intestines) but in addition there are seasonal and regional differences of

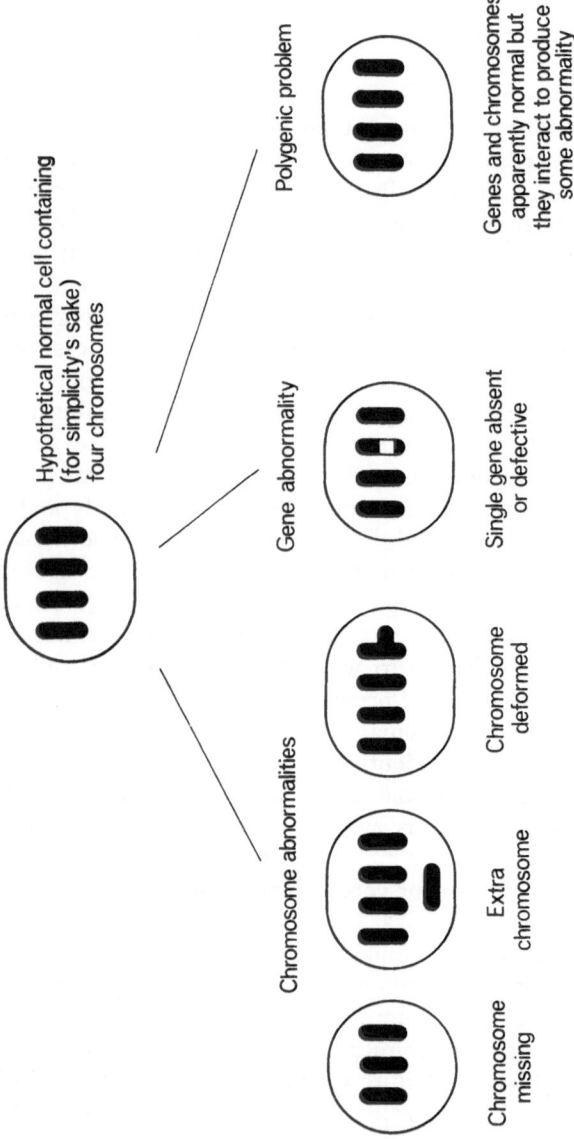

FIG. 31. A simplified diagram showing the range of genetic abnormalities which may be found in man.

incidence that point toward as yet unspecified environmental influences playing a part. Everyone is nowadays aware that German measles (rubella) during early pregnancy may produce congenital changes in eye, ear, heart, or teeth, and that thalidomide given to pregnant women produced many infants with deformed arms or legs. There may be more of such agents of deformity amongst minor infections or chemicals with unsuspected toxicity.

It will emphasize the importance of the difference between disease due to the impact of the environment and intrinsically generated disease to include a portion of a table from a frequently quoted paper (Carter, 1956). This shows the percentage of deaths in a London children's hospital which resulted from environmental and from other causes, mostly genetic, in 1914 and 1954. No doubt the difference would be even more striking in the 1970s.

TABLE 1. *Causes of death (percentage)*

Year	Environmental	Known genetic	Partially genetic and unknown causes
1914	68	2	30
1954	14·5	12	73·5

The diseases which are either directly due to genetic anomaly or are dependent on genetic anomaly if they are to be made manifest by appropriate environmental circumstances can be divided into three relatively distinct groups:

1. Those correlated with visible abnormalities in number or form of chromosomes.

2. Those due to single gene abnormalities.

3. The group referred to earlier where one must assume the interaction of a number of genes—of polygenic origin.

Over-all, about 6 per cent of live-born children show recognizable genetic defects and in rough approximation these are distributed 1:1:4 in groups 1, 2, and 3, respectively.

DISABILITIES ASSOCIATED WITH CHROMOSOMAL
CHANGES

There are relatively large numbers of individuals with chromosomal abnormalities associated with disease in which the diagnosis can be made by the microscopic examination of dividing cells fixed at the right stage (metaphase) of mitosis. These can be obtained either as lymphocytes from the blood or as tissue cells from a fragment of skin. In a properly made slide each dividing nucleus will show 46 chromosomes, including a pair of sex chromosomes which are similar (XX) in the female, different (XY) in the male. The other 22 pairs are known as autosomes and are grouped into classes A–G primarily in accordance with size and numbered 1–22.

As would be expected, any gross abnormality of chromosome number is incompatible with life and it has been stated that as many as 22 per cent of early spontaneous abortions show chromosomal abnormalities which had presumably made the foetus nonviable. Only two groups need be mentioned, sex chromosome anomalies and the 'G-trisomy' anomaly associated with mongolism. There are several anomalous conditions in which X, Y chromosomes are in abnormal combinations such as XO, XXY, XYY, XXX. The type of result can best be seen by comparing the normal male pattern XY with what results when Y is absent (XO) or when there is an additional Y (XYY). Individuals XO are apparent females anatomically but remain sexually immature and are non-fertile. Individuals with XYY have gained some public notoriety recently since it was found that a high proportion of men over 6 ft tall committed to prisons for the criminal insane for murder or other violent crime, showed that abnormality. However, at least two socially normal XYY men have been found. Perhaps one of the most interesting and perplexing problems a paediatrician can face is what to advise about the upbringing of a boy found in some survey to be XYY. At the medico-legal level the existence of such a condition predisposing a person to an antisocial degree of male aggressiveness has an obvious bearing on doctrines of criminal responsibility. No one has yet suggested that any conceivable form of 'genetic engineering' could, by adding X, make an XO intersex into a normal woman, or remove the unwanted Y from the criminal XYY.

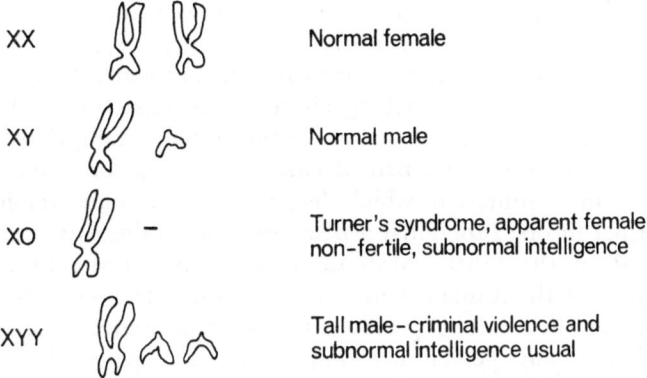

XX		Normal female
XY		Normal male
XO		Turner's syndrome, apparent female non-fertile, subnormal intelligence
XYY		Tall male-criminal violence and subnormal intelligence usual

FIG. 32. Sex chromosome combinations.

Mongolism, now usually spoken of as Down's syndrome to avoid racial implications, is a type of feeble-mindedness with relatively minor anatomical changes seen particularly in children born when their mothers were approaching the menopause. They have 47 chromosomes instead of 46, the additional one being a member of the smallest (G) group of chromosomes. There are 3 instead of 2 examples of chromosome 21, hence the name G-trisomy. The usual explanation is that during the changes which reduce the number of chromosomes from 46 to 23 of the female egg cell, a mechanical error occurs and both the small (no. 21) chromosomes pass to the egg cell instead of one. It has been suggested that ageing may favour such accidents. Another suggestion of great interest has come from Stoller of Melbourne. He finds that in Victoria (south-eastern Australia) there is a wave-like incidence of births of children with Down's syndrome over the years, each peak following an epidemic peak of infectious hepatitis with a lag of nine months. The result has not yet been fully confirmed elsewhere in the world but it raises the possibility that a latent subclinical infection with hepatitis may modify the process of meiosis by which the egg cell is produced.

SINGLE GENE CONDITIONS

Most of the interest in genetic disease has been concentrated on those conditions which depend essentially on alteration of a single gene, allowing a simple Mendelian distribution to appear in the offspring concerned. For fairly obvious reasons, most serious genetic diseases are due to a recessive form of gene. To recapitulate what I said in describing albinism amongst brown-skinned Trobriand islanders, we can make the initial assumption that a certain gene in one of a pair of chromosomes in some individual underwent a mutation which left the chromosome viable but abnormal in one functional aspect. As long as the corresponding gene A in the other chromosome was normal the functional weakness of the mutant gene a was without effect—it was recessive to A. For a long period after the appearance of a in the population, any person carrying it, i.e., Aa genetically, could mate only with normals AA producing equal numbers of Aa and AA children. The frequency of heterozygotes, i.e., of people of Aa type would increase only in parallel with increase in the size of the population as a whole and rather frequently the simple chances of mortality would result in elimination of the gene a from the community. It will become reasonably common only when one or more of three conditions are operative.

1. The same mutation occurs in others with a fairly regular frequency.

2. A small group containing carriers of the gene multiplies freely without outside contacts to produce a large population—the phenomenon of genetic drift.

3. The carriers have a positive survival advantage because of their heterozygous condition.

If there is no such advantage, the accepted rule is that in any large stable freely interbreeding population the mutant gene will reach a proportion where the number of new mutations is equalled by the number of carriers dying without passing on the gene.

The commonest recessive gene in European populations is that associated with cystic fibrosis which is basically a biochemical abnormality of the mucus produced in glands and mucous membranes throughout the body. This results in a variety of disabilities of which undue susceptibility to severe bronchial infections dominates the picture. One in 2,000 children is born with the disease which means, according to Mendel's rule, that four times that number of children are born from $Aa \times Aa$ marriages. This, in turn, means that 1 in 500 marriages in the community are of this character and that 1 in $\sqrt{500}$, i.e., 1:22, 4–5 per cent of all persons carry gene *a* in the heterozygous form *Aa*. Such a high incidence must almost certainly mean that there is some advantage in survival or fertility of the heterozygotes but, so far, the character of that advantage is quite unknown.

There has been an interesting recent development in the understanding of cystic fibrosis. If skin cells from a patient are grown in tissue culture they invariably show a high proportion of cells with granules stained 'metachromatically' with dyes such as toluidine blue. This also holds for parents of such children both of whom are necessarily *Aa*, while amongst random 'normal' individuals, only the expected ± 4 per cent show the reaction. If this should prove a practical test to apply on a large scale it would be theoretically possible to eliminate cystic fibrosis by seeing that all *Aa* individuals mated only with partners certified as *AA*. The other implication now regarded as being of fairly general application is that in the heterozygote (*Aa*) a recessive allele will often produce some minor effect detectable by refined biochemical study.

Two other diseases associated with recessive alleles have features which call for discussion, sickle cell anaemia and phenylketonuria. In the first the heterozygote *Aa* has a survival advantage over *AA* although *aa* is responsible for lethal disease and in phenylketonuria (PKU) a method of ameliorating the *aa* disease has been developed.

Sickle cell anaemia is a rare disease that has been studied almost exclusively in American Negroes. It is a severe and usually fatal anaemia and derives its name from the shape the red cells take when examined under the microscope. The parents of such a child show no anaemia but they also have detectable changes in their blood and are heterozygous *Aa* for the gene *a* which in double dose, can produce the severe disease. These heterozygotes are said to show sickle cell trait. Since Pauling showed that there were two different haemoglobins present in the red cells of persons with sickle cell trait, the topic of sickle cell haemoglobin and its evolutionary implications has become the showpiece in the shop-window of molecular biology. Here is a lethal disease dependent on a point-mutation in a single gene which changed one amino acid in the haemoglobin *A* chain from glutamic acid to valine and no more. In many ways this represented the beginning of molecular genetics. Once the way had been opened, a large range of other mutants of human haemoglobin were found, though none of them were as common or as significant for biological theory as the gene Hb^s the official equivalent of what in this context I have called *a*.

When something excitingly new appears in their field, scientists have a habit of finding that they had more spare time than they had imagined and in a big way or a small way 'hopping on to the bandwagon'. People interested in blood group work or the distribution of serum proteins in the different races of Africa extended their interests to check on haemoglobin S. It was not long before a map of Africa could be drawn to show the percentage distribution of Hb^s, i.e., of the sickle cell trait in people of the various regions. It was as high as 40 per cent in one or two regions of Central Africa and showed a belt with more than 10 per cent over most of rain-forested tropical Africa. This corresponded essentially to the region where malaria is heavily prevalent. The obvious deduction was that in a malarial environment it is an advantage to have the sickle cell trait, and the evidence reported does indicate that infections with malignant tertian malaria, particularly in young children, are less severe in the heterozygous than in those with normal haemoglobin. Since the malarial parasite multiplies in the red cell living largely on haemoglobin, it is not surprising that this should be so. If there are 10 per cent of the population carrying the gene Hb^s amongst these there will be thirty-nine Aa's with a relative resistance to malaria for every one with the virtually lethal combination aa. If the mortality from malaria in childhood is high and the benefit of being heterozygous rather than normal is significant, then clearly the population can carry the inevitable mortality of aa's and show a net advantage.

The fact that populations with significant concentrations of people with sickle cell trait are found only in malarial regions is the most striking verification of the principles of population genetics available in man. It is rare, however, for a mutation of a single gene to provide a change which either in the heterozygote or homozygote confers a positive survival advantage and, apart from another gene, responsible for a different type of anaemia in Mediterranean countries (thalassaemia) with a similar probable relation to malaria, no other examples are known. Perhaps the

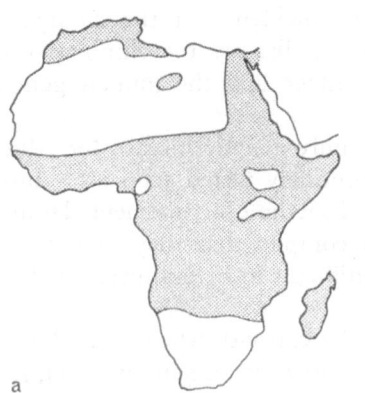

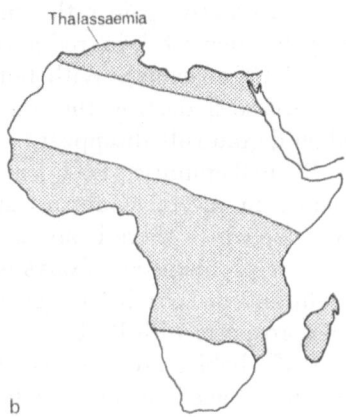

a   b

FIG. 33. Maps of Africa showing:
(a) the distribution of malaria before
modern control measures came into
operation; (b) the distribution of abnormal haemoglobins which are
thought to provide some resistance to
malaria. (Note that the haemoglobin
abnormality which occurs along the
North African Coast is known as
thalassaemia while that which occurs
in other parts is known as sickle cell
haemoglobin.) (c) The distribution of
Burkitt lymphoma (note that there
are areas within this distribution—
cold or hot—where the tumour is
rare, but there are no areas outside
the distribution where the tumour is
known to be common).

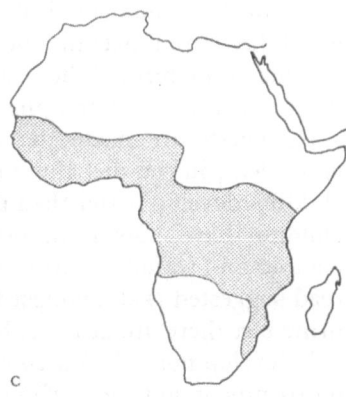

c

most interesting feature of thalassaemia is that in Italian districts where *Aa* heterozygotes are common, up to 20 per cent, and can be recognized by blood examination, marriage counselling services to warn against the marriage of *Aa* with *Aa* have been largely successful in reducing the incidence of the *aa* disease (Cooley's anaemia). With both these diseases the elimination of malaria will destroy the *Aa* advantage and the mutant gene *a* should gradually disappear.

Phenylketonuria (PKU) is the only genetic disease for which babies in several countries are routinely tested soon after birth and for which there is an accepted method of treatment. Human genetic problems are always more complex than they seem at first sight and in 1971 it has become difficult to be enthusiastic about the prospects with PKU.

PKU babies are born lacking the capacity to convert phenylalanine, one of the amino acids essential for human nutrition, into tyrosine, the next stage in its normal process of metabolism. There results an abnormally high concentration of phenylalanine in the blood and a high excretion of an abnormal product, a phenyl ketone in the urine. If a high concentration of phenylalanine persists over the first few years of life there is serious brain damage and many such children become low-grade mental defectives. It is theoretically simple to deal with such a disease. Design a diet which has a minimal amount of phenylalanine and feed the infant on this from birth. There are available digests of milk protein from which most of the phenylalanine is chemically removed. If such digests are made the main source of protein, or protein equivalent, in the diet there is no doubt that a proportion of the children develop better than the average untreated case. But many children have now been detected and treated in one way or another and serious doubts are being expressed. The last paper I read suggested that amongst the infants that give a positive PKU urine test there are at least three groups, some whose intelligence will develop normally on conventional diet, some who do no good on treatment and some who do well. In some, the lowering of the level of phenylalanine which can be tolerated in the blood is highly critical. Too much gives brain damage, too little gives a condition that resembles a protein deficiency disease well known in African children under the name kwashiorkor, and itself giving rise to brain damage. Some children with dangerously high phenylalanine amounts in the blood give a negative urine test.

It is still orthodox paediatric practice that a PKU baby should be treated but from the humanitarian point of view it is hard to assess how much it is worth. But it will probably be many years before the logical solution can be accepted that infants with gross genetic defects of metabolism should be treated as those with no brain (anencephalic monsters) or other gross anatomical distortions are treated today and not allowed to survive.

THE DIFFICULTIES OF GENETIC ENGINEERING

In Chapter 4 I discussed in general terms the widely accepted suggestion that 'genetic engineering' was a possibility of the future—that some day a faulty gene could be replaced by a normal one. I discussed the possibility, perhaps in too cavalier a fashion, as something which would remain for ever impossible to apply to actual human individuals with genetic disease. To wind up this account of some of the genetic diseases to which it might be applied, I felt that I should restate the difficulties in more specific fashion.

Let us look then at what would be involved in attempting to introduce a 'good' gene into a patient suffering from some double recessive condition like PKU or cystic fibrosis. This is based on the finding that fragments of host DNA can be caught into virus particles during their final stages of construction and if the virus is a temperate one, allowing continuing survival and multiplication of the host cells the segment of DNA being carried may be incorporated into a new host. When this occurs in a bacterial virus the process is known as transduction. There is evidence that the temperate animal virus polyoma can take up mouse DNA from tissue culture cells and that some of the visible virus particles (virions) are pseudo-virions with *only* mouse DNA. They are therefore incapable of multiplication but could in principle ferry new genes into the next cell entered by the virion. Evidence for such actions is derived wholly from tissue culture studies arranged so that the situation comes as close as possible to the bacteriological set up required to demonstrate the transduction of bacterial genetic characters by bacterial viruses.

The procedure envisaged to cure a PKU baby would be approximately as follows: First, the structure of the normal human enzyme E responsible for the primary oxidation of phenylalanine to tyrosine must be established, in itself a task of considerable difficulty mainly because of the difficulty of obtaining enough of the *human* enzyme. If this is an average-sized protein with 300 amino acid units the task of obtaining the correct sequence with limited supplies of raw material would be considerable. The next step would be to synthesize chemically the double-stranded DNA that controls synthesis of the enzyme, each strand of about 1,000 nucleotides. Even if one strand would be adequate as a template on which to base biological synthesis *in vitro* this is far beyond current achievement although probably within the range of the physically possible, if adequate motivation and unlimited funds were available. Once the pattern had been laid down, replicated by the enzymatic techniques of Kornberg's school and its capacity to produce enzyme E *in vitro* verified, the real difficulties begin. We have, it will be assumed, unlimited amounts of the gene available in solution. What is needed is to 'cure' the cells responsible for production of enzyme E—at a guess, all or a proportion of liver cells—which now carry genes which, owing to mutation, produce a protein similar to E but lacking the effective molecular configuration. The need is for incorporation of the gene into an appropriate virus which is known to invade human liver cells without producing hepatitis or, more slowly, malignant disease. I can see no possible way by which a virus could be found or developed with that combination of qualities nor, if it existed, can I see any way by which its possession of the required qualities for use in PKU babies could ever be proved to the satisfaction of a Food and Drug Administration or any other responsible authority. The next difficulty is that having regard to the character of virus multiplication and the existence of enzymes splitting DNA in the cell, there seems to be no way of getting gene E into the virus that would be more successful than simply growing the virus on a human tissue line known to be able to produce enzyme E, though necessarily in only minute amount. Finally having, we assume, overcome the difficulty of charging the virus with the right gene and ensuring that it has the right virulence and no more, so that it can enter at least a majority of liver cells and unload the gene it carries inside the nucleus, we face the most difficult problem of all. How does the gene find its right place in a quiescent nucleus, oust the abnormal gene and incorporate itself, lined up correctly, in the place left vacant? The answer is the same as before. At every step, one can with some hesitation say that with the rather restricted knowledge we have, this may be possible in principle but the practical problems would take an army of first-rate scientists and technicians to overcome them. There could never, in my opinion, be adequate motivation for any government to finance such a research or for any individual scientist to undertake the responsibility of its technical direction.

THE ETHICS OF GENETIC MEDICINE

I read a good deal about paediatric research and I find it intensely characteristic of the present stage of medical science, and profoundly disquieting, that the best research being done in the great children's hospitals of the world is mostly concerned with genetic abnormalities in infants. To an enthusiastic biochemist or immunologist, rare genetic abnormalities in infants can provide fascinating opportunities to get a clearer understanding of some of the minutiae of living process which can be gained in no other way. If he is successful he may well be able to devise some strictly controlled regimen which will keep the child alive but grossly handicapped and with no prospect of a normal existence.

As an immunologist I have been especially interested in the range of rare anomalies whereby in one way or another a child cannot deal with infection in normal fashion. Thirty years ago all such children 'failed to thrive' and died early from common or obscure infections. With the coming of the antibiotics, some of these children were saved and in 1952 it was recognized that in one such condition the children had no gamma globulin, which is the protein fraction of the blood that contains all the antibodies needed for dealing with bacterial infection. This condition of 'congenital sex-linked agammaglobulinaemia' occurs only in boys. Its detailed study has had a most important influence on the development of our understanding of defence processes in the body and in fact was very largely responsible for the acceptance of the concept of the two immune systems that I described in Chapter 1. To recapitulate briefly in the present context, the thymus-dependent or T-system of cell-mediated immunity is the more primitive. Its function is to produce and mobilize cells (immunocytes) with specialized defence functions for dealing primarily with foreign cells. The cells may be recognized as foreign either because they *are* foreign (transplants) or because they have been modified by somatic mutation, by virus action or by taking up of certain chemical substances. The second thymus-independent or B-system functions by producing antibody from proliferated clones of plasma cells. It may be useful to think of antibody as an antiseptic designed to kill just one sort of bacteria while the T-cells are also of many different types, each of which will recognize and react with only one type of foreign or altered cell.

It was largely because in children with the genetic abnormality, agammaglobulinaemia, the whole activity of the B—antibody-producing—system was switched off, that it became possible to understand clearly the important, and till then largely unappreci-ated, role of the second system of cell-mediated immunity.

This was very gratifying to scholarly immunologists but the human side had its tragedies. Before antibiotics, such children died from pneumonia as soon as they lost the temporary antibody and immunity they had received from their mother's blood. With meticulous nursing care, the early use of antibiotics for any infection, and regular doses of ready-made antibody in the form of purified gamma globulin from normal human blood, the children can be kept in fairly good health. The first child so treated in the late 1940s was reported in 1967 as being still well on a dose of gamma globulin every month, with an excellent job as cashier in a bank in Norfolk, Virginia. Others have not been so fortunate. Several have died from hepatitis and a few, but still a vastly greater proportion than in normal young people, have developed malignant disease of the lymph glands. Many suffer from joint trouble closely related to rheumatoid arthritis.

The story in its own way is rather like that of the PKU babies. If the paediatrician is wise and well informed and is lucky in that his patient is a typical case with no minor or major genetic anoma-lies elsewhere to complicate the position, then he may be able to provide a tolerable life for the child by the orthodox treatment. I have no figures, but from the literature one gathers that full success in either group is rare, there are many failures and some-times well-meant treatment can do serious harm. Another aspect which must not be emphasized unduly but which must not be forgotten is the very great expense to the community of treating the metabolic and immunological deficiencies of infants which would otherwise be lethal. Much of that expense may be absorbed initially in research budgets but research programmes do not go on for ever. Once a child has survived to an age where he can have some insight into his own condition and some understanding and fear of death, there is a moral obligation on the research team or the community to continue the treatment necessary for survival at any cost. This is the stage at which all concerned may feel that it was neither moral nor humanitarian to have intervened at all in a hopeless situation.

CONGENITAL MALFORMATIONS

Congenital malformations have already been mentioned briefly as having both genetic and environmental factors in their causation. They are common conditions whose existence is known to everyone, and since time immemorial Omar Khayyam's question, 'What did the Hand then of the Potter shake?' has been asked. The modern answer to that question still fails to satisfy. An expert group discussing the matter for the World Health Organization decided that a polygenic type of genetic component was involved, the expression of which could be modified by factors of the foetal environment whose nature was still unknown. It is an answer without any significant impact on prediction or prevention of any specific type of malformation.

Three may be taken for further brief discussion, congenital pyloric stenosis, spina bifida, and anencephaly, mainly in relation to the practical and ethical aspects of how the victims are treated.

On the surface, congenital pyloric stenosis is one of the success stories of paediatrics. An experienced paediatrician can recognize the symptoms within a few weeks of birth and a simple operation to divide a hypertrophied band of muscle which prevents the stomach from emptying into the duodenum, will usually leave the child essentially normal for the rest of its life. Here there is no ethical problem whatever. The condition must be recognized as early as possible and dealt with surgically. The risk that such infants when they grow up will have children with the same condition, is small but it is significantly larger than for unaffected individuals. Statistical study of the incidence of pyloric stenosis according to sex show a 5:1 preponderance in males. Close relatives such as siblings or children of an index case show a higher incidence and if the index case is a female there is a considerably larger incidence of cases in relatives than is the case with the commoner male index case.

Very much the same can be said about harelip and cleft palate, congenital dislocation of the hip, and various types of club-foot. All have a genetic component and a possible but, as yet undiscovered, effect of the foetal environment. A tolerable and sometimes an excellent anatomical and functional repair can be looked forward to after skilled surgical treatment.

Spina bifida is a failure of the lower part of the spinal cord to develop normally. It is a distressing and usually lethal complaint which has challenged surgeons to attempt reconstructive and palliative operations. With intensive care and special attention to the prevention of infection, such children can be kept alive but there is a growing feeling that the effort cannot be justified.

Anencephaly is probably due to a rather similar failure of development in the embryonic tube which develops into the central nervous system but here it involves the upper end and the brain fails to develop. The infant may be born alive but there is no brain, the head ends behind the face with no cranial vault. It is a repulsive and frightening object and the orthodox handling of the situation is to give the 'monstrous birth' an injection of morphia and make no effort for its survival. So we find ourselves having to look firmly at one of the aspects of the human situation that is usually relegated to the unconscious as something cruel, unjust, and altogether inexplicable and unpreventable.

I started with the problem of inter-racial differences of intelligence and other mental qualities and to what extent they were of genetic origin. The answer is almost certainly that genetic factors are responsible for 80 per cent of the differences between children who are otherwise healthy and have had broadly similar upbringing, but that, when we cannot make those two last statements, we can only guess that genetic factors are still the most important.

I was particularly interested to read a summing up of the situation by an experienced field anthropologist with a special interest in disease patterns in primitive society (Gajdusek, 1968). He warned against the implicit assumption in much work in cultural anthropology, that each member of the group has essentially the same neurological equipment as a genetic endowment and that behavioural differences between groups are of wholly cultural origin. Probably the feature on which Gajdusek wished to lay most emphasis was the diversity of gross structural differences between individual brains whenever the necessarily elaborate studies were made. Quite large differences involving mid-brain nuclei, structure of the frontal lobe, etc., were found between individual brains from New Guinea subjects and there can be no doubt that many finer structural differences were present. Gajdusek then lists the extremely wide range of damaging circumstances that can modify development before and during birth, all of them more likely to affect primitive peoples than Western populations. Maternal infections (rubella, syphilis, etc.) trauma, nutritional deficiencies, endocrine disease, and exposure to toxic substances may all damage the foetus. Attempts at abortion and primitive obstetrical practices, as well as the normal hazards of birth trauma, must be considered. Most infectious diseases are experienced during childhood; mild or severe neurological complications are common and there are strong suspicions that brain involvement, notably in measles, can interfere with intellectual development. Gajdusek also notes the multiform effects on behaviour and intelligence of chronic iodine lack and cretinism, which may affect whole communities as in the Western Highlands of New Guinea.

A man's temperament, social behaviour, and specific skills are all shaped by his cultural environment but their quality will be influenced, sometimes overwhelmingly, by his genetic inheritance, by damage sustained before and during birth and by a variety of accidental non-cultural damage, notably from infections, during childhood.

7

TOWARDS PROGRESS IN CANCER

To a great many people, medically trained scientists as well as laymen, the pot of gold at the end of the rainbow of medical research is the discovery of the cause and cure of cancer. It is a current article of faith that if America can put a man on the Moon, America can discover the cause of cancer. In Arizona there is, we are told, a cemetery where people who have died of cancer are preserved by being frozen in liquid nitrogen 'in the sure and certain hope' of revival and cure by the medical scientists of the twenty-first or twenty-second century. I have been and remain a sceptic and was castigated in public by a local president of the British Medical Association for saying about ten years ago that I could see no hope for any revolutionary improvement in the cure of cancer. It is still an unpopular attitude. As long as money for research must be sought from men without sophisticated understanding of biology we can be certain that every geneticist and molecular biologist will be careful to add to his exposition of what he is doing, the safely irrefutable statement that it may well have importance for the understanding of cancer!

Perhaps it is wise to start with a brief outline of the nature of cancer as it was known to physicians and pathologists of the late nineteenth century in the days before cancer research in its modern sense had even begun. Yet in 1890, say, clinical observation, analysis of post-mortem findings, and simple types of microscopic study had made the outline of cancer clear. A cancer was a mass of proliferating body cells that seemed to have escaped from the constraints which kept all other cells of the body in proper place and function. The proliferation ate into neighbouring tissues and ulcerated through the skin. Often cells with the insane capacity for growth slipped loose from the tumour and lodged in lymph gland, lung, liver, or elsewhere to produce secondary tumours or metastases. Unless surgery could remove the tumour completely before such secondary spread had taken place, death was inevitable.

It was known to everyone that cancer was predominantly a disease of old age but there were differences of detail in the pattern of age incidence for cancer in different sites. It was known, too, that certain sites were much commoner than others; breast, stomach, uterus, and prostate predominated then; lung cancer is very much a twentieth-century disease. Clinical observation long ago made it clear that chronic local irritation could result in cancer. Smokers of clay pipes suffered from cancer of the lower lip, persons chronically exposed to soot or lubricating oil showed special forms of cancer that became known as chimney sweeps' or mule spinners' cancers in nineteenth-century England. Not very many years after the introduction of X-rays to medicine it became obvious that skin cancer of the hands was an occupational hazard of radiologists. One has only to add to these real observations the myth of 'cancer houses' in which successive occupiers were specially prone to die of cancer to find a suggestion that cancer might be an infectious disease. Such findings provided the ideas which could be worked on in the laboratories as the experimental phase of cancer study began.

EXPERIMENTAL CANCER RESEARCH

Research on cancer has attracted almost every great medical scientist from Paul Ehrlich to Albert Sabin and it is essential to have an outline of how research on cancer developed if we are to understand its limitations. The first objective of experimental work was, of course, to find a suitable form of cancer in a laboratory animal which could be obtained with some regularity.

Initially it was necessary to rely on the spontaneous appearance of malignant disease in mice or rats which were approaching the end of their life span. Very soon, however, the hints from clinical experience were applied in the laboratory to make the deliberate induction of cancer in experimental animals, particularly mice, a routine procedure.

By 1915 it was known that rabbits' ears painted with tar developed warts and then cancer, and that irradiation of animals with X-rays would accelerate the appearance of tumours. In 1911, Rous had discovered a sarcoma (a type of cancer) of birds which could be transmitted by filtered material and was therefore probably caused by a virus.

The use of tar to produce skin cancer provided an attractive field for chemists to collaborate with pathologists and the isolation of the responsible chemicals (polycyclic hydrocarbons) was the the first major success in cancer research. Early in the work, mice had replaced rabbits as the most convenient experimental animal. Large numbers could be painted at regular intervals with any substance to be tested and the results were easily read and reproducible. Soon the chemists had synthesized many related chemicals of high cancer-producing power. Some of these, such as MCA (methylcholanthrene), to be mentioned later, have become standard reagents for cancer investigation.

The main physical agent used in experimental cancer work was and has remained irradiation, first with X-rays and later from radio-isotopes either as a distant source of gamma-rays or by implantation in some part of the body.

The approach to cancer as an infectious disease was opened up by Peyton Rous in 1911 but it tells a good deal, to say that Rous shared a Nobel prize for this discovery in 1967, fifty-six years later. Only when the easily handled 'cancer viruses' of mice became available in the 1950s did the opinion develop that cancer might turn out to be 'a virus disease'. Polyoma virus of mice, discovered in 1956, was specially impressive in the way that on inoculation into newborn mice or hamsters *multiple* tumours were produced. By 1960, therefore, there were available convenient ways by which malignant tumours could be regularly produced in experimental animals by the application of physical or chemical carcinogens or by injection of 'oncogenic', i.e., cancer-producing, viruses.

An advance of almost greater importance for cancer research had emerged rather slowly in the 1940s—the use of 'pure line mice'. With the development of genetics it became clear that all animals were heterozygous and that even litter mates could differ in genetic characteristics. Theoretically it was also evident that by a prolonged series of brother–sister matings it should be possible to sort out from any standard mixed population of mice, animal lines which were homozygous for almost all genes. Many such lines were of low fertility or congenitally unsuitable in one way or another but with the equivalent of the horticulturists' 'green fingers', experienced mouse breeders could produce robust pure line mice, some strains of which, such as 'C3H' or 'C57Bl', are maintained in almost every biological laboratory in the world. Experimental cancer research provided much of the incentive for this work. One of the first objectives was to obtain 'high cancer' or 'high leukaemia' strains, i.e., mice which could be relied upon to show, say, a high spontaneous incidence of breast cancer, or mice which almost all developed lymphatic leukaemia by the time they were a year old. Such strains were obtained and opened up important new lines of research.

Another virtue of pure line mice also became apparent. With the old standard strains, tumours appeared in old mice but only rarely could they be transferred to normal mice of the same colony. When a tumour arose in a pure line mouse a fragment of the tumour implanted into a young animal of the same line 'took' with ease and grew into a large tumour of the same character as that from which it was derived. The process of transfer could be continued indefinitely but only so long as the work was done wholly within the same pure line strain.

The next major line of advance was the recognition of the influence of hormones on cancer. The function of breast, uterus, and prostate—three notable areas of cancer in man—is largely controlled by hormone action. Collaboration between endocrinologists and cancer workers soon provided fascinating examples of malignant tumours which could be made to wither away by appropriate hormonal manipulations and others which could be called into existence by hormone overaction. The artificial female sex hormone, stilboestrol, is widely applied in the treatment of cancer of the prostate in man and a variety of procedures to reduce hormonal activity such as surgical removal of the pituitary gland have sometimes been successful in holding back advanced breast cancer with secondary deposits elsewhere in the body. The impressions one obtains from extensive reading in this field are, first, the intimidating complexity of the interactions of different hormones in the body; second, the wide variability of tumours in the same organ in their response to hormone therapy; and third, the temporary nature of the majority of the favourable results obtained in the hormonal treatment of human cancer.

The most recent experimental development and the only one on which I have myself written extensively is the recognition that immune response against tumours is possible. One of my chief interests in the last five years has been in developing the concept of 'immunological surveillance'. The gist of this is that one of the main functions of the complex mechanisms that have been uncovered by immunological research is to police the body for any abnormal mutant cells which by developing toward malignancy threaten survival. That is perhaps not more than a speculative extension from the facts and, as yet, no significant practical application of the antigenic quality of tumours to the treatment of cancer has been developed.

The last area of research to be mentioned is the search for drugs specifically active against cancer and leukaemia which is essentially cancer of the white blood cells. If we exclude hormones and synthetic drugs of similar structure, the anti-cancer drugs all act by virtue of the fact that actively multiplying cells are more vulnerable to many poisons than quiescent cells. The processes of DNA duplication and mitosis, that complex ballet of the chromosomes by which one nucleus becomes two, require many specialized enzyme actions susceptible to interference by chemical agents. There are now a number of chemicals known to interfere with defined parts of the process of protein synthesis that was described in Chapter 2 and others, including most of those used in cancer treatment with generally similar but less clearly definable effects. Every anti-cancer drug also has a harmful effect on multiplying normal cells and it is not surprising that a number of these drugs are carcinogenic in normal animals in the sense that when applied specifically for that purpose they can provoke cancer. This is not necessarily a serious objection to their use in conditions which would otherwise be rapidly fatal. In the acute leukaemias of childhood appropriate drugs can give a consistent prolongation of life sometimes for five years or more but no one has yet claimed permanent elimination of the disease.

I have enumerated eight major areas of experimental research on cancer. Every one has been and is being widely studied and wherever suitable leads have been recognized, clinical applications have been attempted. One can, however, still sum up the consensus of medical opinion in three rules:

1. Recognize the existence of cancer as early as possible.

2. Remove the malignant tissue as completely as possible by surgery.

3. Use X-rays to deal with any small numbers of cancer cells that have escaped surgical removal.

The appropriate parts to be played by surgery and irradiation in any given case will always need intelligent decision by surgeon and radiologist but their basis of decision will be an empirical one based on clinical experience.

Experimental research has so far had few directly practical results, hormone therapy and drug treatment have in general been used only when the orthodox methods cannot be applied or after they have failed. There is no more fascinating area of biological study than laboratory research in cancer and there is probably no section of it which cannot occasionally provide hints that may improve the treatment of some individual patient. One cannot, however, avoid a sense of disappointment. Why has the outcome of sixty years' work by many first-rate scientists and at a cost of hundreds of millions of dollars, had so insignificant an influence on the prevention or treatment of cancer? The rest of this chapter is concerned with an attempt to answer this question.

IS THERE A 'CAUSE' OF CANCER?

In the first instance we can concentrate upon what, after all, is the basic question of the origin of malignant disease. One might ask simply, What causes cancer? but for reasons which I hope will become clear I should prefer to put the question as, what are the conditions associated with the emergence of cancer in man? I believe that one of the main misconceptions of the cancerous process springs from the concern of most workers in cancer research to seek and find external 'causes' for cancer.

There is no question that one can legitimately speak of the inoculation of polyoma virus into newborn mice, heavy cigarette smoking in man, or the feeding of certain organic chemicals to rats as 'causing cancer'. The concept of causation here is, however, very different from what is applied to the cause of measles or a broken limb. Using cancer for any type of malignant cellular proliferation occurring in man we can make a number of statements which are highly relevant to its understanding.

1. A cancer cell is an actively functioning cell capable of indefinite proliferation under adequate conditions and maintaining its charac-

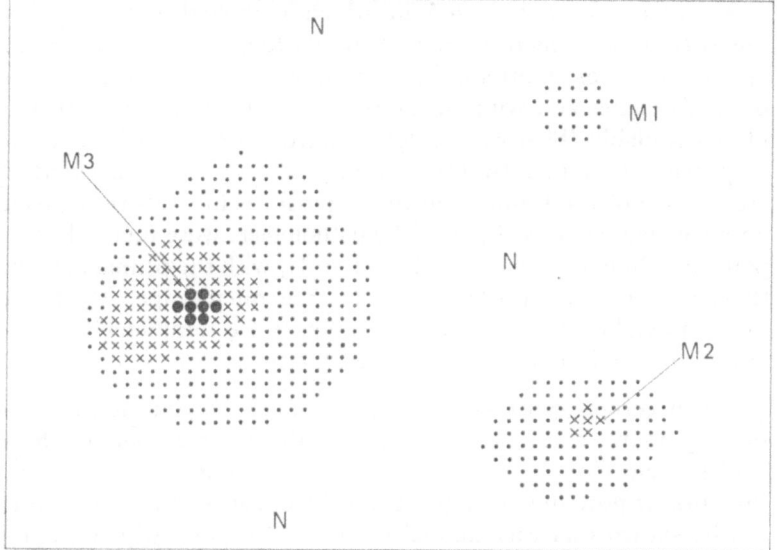

F I G. 34. To illustrate the concepts of sequential somatic mutation and the monoclonal origin of cancer. • = first mutation; × = second mutation; ● = third mutation (malignant change). Each mutation has a proliferative advantage over the preceding cell type, from which it rises, and grows at the expense of the original cell population indicated by the empty background N.

teristics by inheritance. In the period of its first appearance as cancer the process of nuclear division (mitosis) takes place normally. The only essential abnormality of the cell is its capacity to proliferate in abnormal fashion within the body.

2. Under certain circumstances it is possible to decide that all the cells of a given cancer are descendants of a single cell. Perhaps the most important finding to be established about cancer in general is that many tumours and malignant conditions of the blood cells are *mono-clonal*, that is, they give every indication that the tumour started from *one* cell. This has been shown for myelocytic leukaemia, myelomatosis, and macroglobulinaemia amongst the blood cell cancers and for uterine myoma (a benign tumour) and Burkitt lymphoma.

3. Probably related to 2 is the fact known to all experienced pathologists that any tumour has its own individuality of microscopic structure.

A test has been reported in which pathologists were given microscopic sections from each of twenty lung cancers removed at operation or post-mortem. This was a standard set labelled with patient's names and with all the relevant data about the patient's illness available. That was straightforward. The test took the form of providing another twenty sections, each representing another area of one of the tumours in the original set but this time given only a coded label, A, B, etc. The pathologists were then asked to pair each slide, with their labels A, B to U, with the primary set on the basis of their appearance under the microscope. Most got fifteen to eighteen 'right'. No two tumours are completely alike— at the somatic level they are genetically different.

4. When certain cancer-producing chemicals are injected appropriately in mice or guinea-pigs, e.g., the hydrocarbon methylcholanthrene (MCA), 80 or 90 per cent of the animals will produce tumours. If pure line, i.e., genetically identical animals, are used it can be shown that each animal produces a tumour which is antigenically different from that arising in any other animal of the group.

The four qualities, all of them unequivocally established, only make sense on one interpretation—that the essential starting-point of any cancer is a single cell. That is a definite statement but it should be considered carefully for what it does not mean, as well as for what it does. We know that once a cancer has appeared and is kept alive, either by natural transplantation to another part of the patient's body (metastasis) or by artificial transplantation into experimental animals of the same pure strain, inheritable differences from the original cancer are almost certain to become evident. A very common result is to find a visible change in the number of chromosomes in each cell and in experimental cancers a greater ease of transfer to a new recipient animal. One may deduce from this the possibility that it may take more than one mutational change for a cell to become malignant. It is also by no means excluded that when a tumour arises in an irritated area, such as the bronchial tree of a heavy cigarette smoker, more than one 'ancestral' cancer cell may be involved.

At the risk of over-emphasizing the point of the single cell origin of malignant disease, I want to return here to one of the features of somatic mutation which I discussed in an earlier chapter. Somatic mutation, being a *rare* inheritable change in a single body

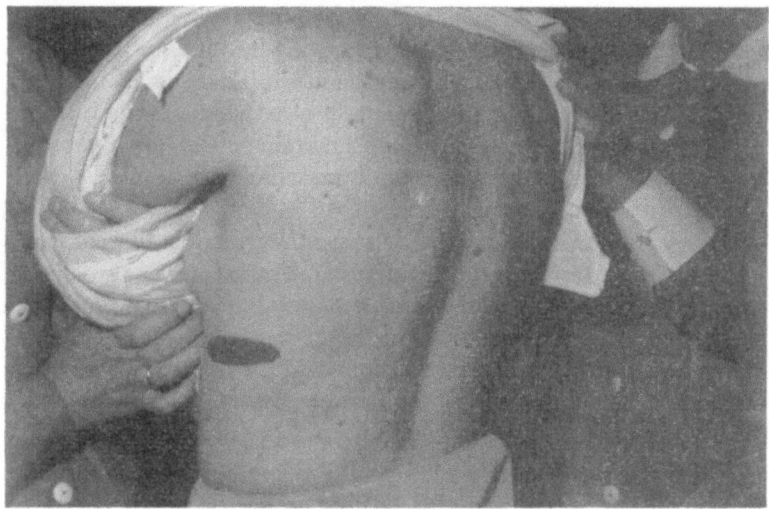

F IG. 35. A birthmark: a somatic mutation in a melanocyte occurring in embryonic life. (By courtesy of Dr E. M. Nichols.)

cell, will have no visible or functionally demonstrable result unless the change induced by mutation can be magnified by active proliferation of the mutant cell concerned. Perhaps the simplest example to understand is a birthmark on the skin, a brown mole ranging in size from a mere freckle to a patch an inch or two across. Each represents a mutation of one of the melanocytes— the pigment cells that lodge in the superficial layer of the skin— a mutation that took place at some period of embryonic life. The larger the birthmark the earlier the initiating mutation took place.

When a somatic cell in an adult mutates, it will remain wholly inconspicuous unless as a result of the mutation it is, either intrinsically or as a result of some hormonal stimulus, provoked to proliferate more actively than other cells in its particular tissue or cell community. The proliferation may be quite benign. Any one over 60 has only to look at the back of his hands to see a variety of brown spots and an occasional warty thickening of the skin (hyperkeratoses) which are certainly the result of somatic mutation plus proliferation of the mutant cell. Malignancy (cancer) is really a rather wide term to cover any proliferative process that actually invades adjacent or distant tissues of the body. Cancer is not a unitary disease like measles or tuberculosis. It is a manifestation of abnormal proliferative growth by the descendants of a mutant cell, a clone of cells which, for any one of a hundred or a thousand reasons, has escaped from normal control. There is an intensely random character about malignant disease which I can best express by saying that it results when a certain cell *happens* to undergo a change in its genetic structure which *happens to* give it capacity for abnormal proliferation.

This is merely another way of saying that the quantitative study of cancer must be based on the fact that it is essentially a stochastic process, random but with statistical regularities, which I have already contrasted with determinative processes where there is a clear quantitative relationship between cause and effect. The differences are not absolute. No matter how strictly determined a process seems to be, a 'random scatter' appears whenever we try to measure to the limit of accuracy the relation between cause and effect. Equally the 'random regularities' of stochastic processes are only regular when they are not distorted by changing conditions. This is specially relevant to the understanding of cancer.

Cigarettes and lung cancer

There is not the slightest doubt about the importance of heavy cigarette smoking as a 'cause' of cancer of the lung in the sense that if cigarette smoking stopped today there would be first a slowing down of the current progressive increase in lung cancer deaths, then perhaps in fifteen to twenty years' time a rapid fall in the number of deaths, to a small fraction of the present numbers. But it would not be to zero. Equally, whenever I have been crusading against cigarettes, I have always had to be honest and say that 80 per cent of heavy smokers will *not* get lung cancer. The basis for these statements can be seen in the graph (Fig. 36) which shows the lung cancer incidence at each five-year age period for males born in successive decades since 1860–70. Each such group is known to statisticians as a cohort, and we can be sure that each cohort up to the present has, during its adult period, comprised a progressively increasing number of cigarette smokers. It is characteristic of stochastic processes of the type concerned with cancer to give a straight-line graph of age incidence when plotted in the fashion I have used in the graph. The significant feature is that the lines for each cohort are nearly straight lines and are not far from being parallel. In each, the rules for a stochastic process hold. But

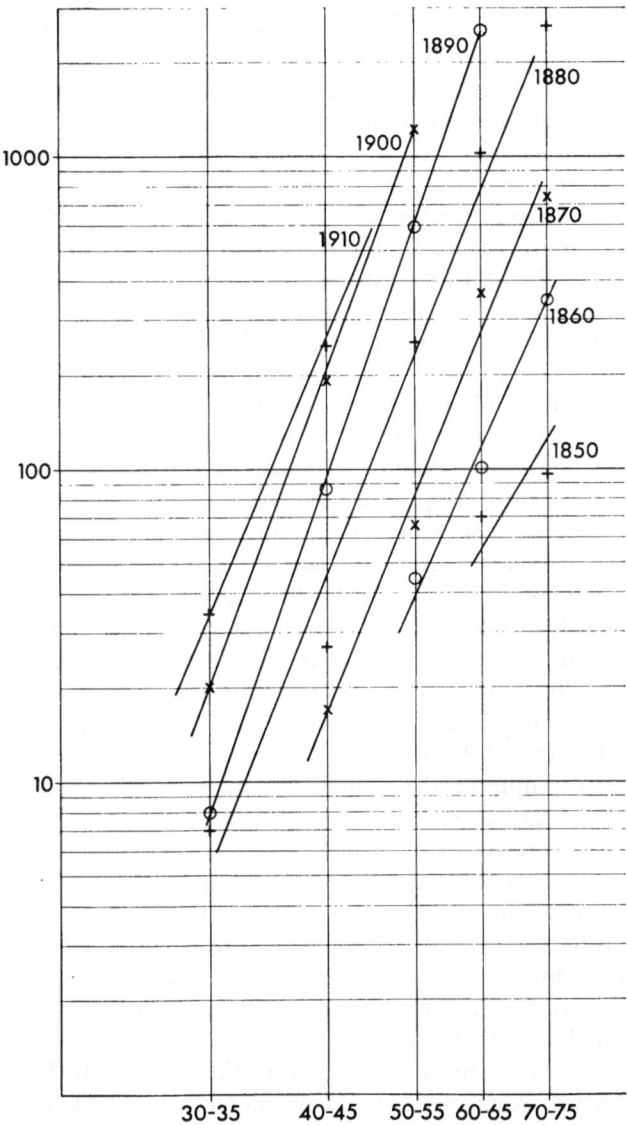

F IG. 36. Age-specific incidence of death from lung cancer according to date of birth (males, England and Wales). To show the approximate straight lines when figures for deaths per million per annum and age are both plotted on logarithmic scales. Note how for each successive group the line is shifted to the left but all remain approximately parallel.

the line moves to the left for each successive cohort as lung cancer occurs more frequently at each age. It is this movement to the left that gives an indication and a measure of the increasing consumption of cigarettes and the larger proportion of men who smoke them.

There are many possible irritants in cigarette smoke, including tarry substances, and the effects on the lining of the bronchial tubes are complex and include varying degrees of proliferation of the lining cells from which cancerous mutants can arise. When the bronchial tubes are examined post-mortem from heavy smokers who have *not* died of lung cancer, a wide range of cell proliferation below but often coming close to malignant level, can be seen. It is probably impossible to say what is the exact nature of these pre-malignant changes but there is no doubt whatever that they provide a large population of cells that are predisposed to undergo the mutation that will produce a definite cancer.

The tobacco companies have consistently claimed that the evidence against cigarettes was 'wholly statistical'. The statement is quite true but it is equally true for every generalization that has ever been legitimately made about a complex human situation. The incrimination of the cigarette in vastly increasing the incidence of lung cancer, is at least as well established as the efficacy of Salk vaccine against polio or that the elimination of malaria lowers the general death-rate of a tropical country.

As an example of the complexity of the situation where the initiation of cancer is concerned and still keeping to the general theme of cigarettes and cancer, one can mention some recent findings of the effect of other lung irritants. Workers exposed to asbestos fibres in the air, and uranium miners who are liable to inhale repeatedly small amounts of radioactive gas, both have excessively high rates of lung cancer—but the excess is confined to men who are also heavy cigarette smokers. Then there is the well-established fact that lung cancer in heavy cigarette smokers is more frequent in city dwellers than in those living in the country although urban smog produces no increase in non-smokers. All three findings underline the predisposition to lung cancer induced by cigarette smoking.

Before leaving the question of how chemical substances are responsible for the initiation of cancer, one must pay some consideration to the fact that of the many thousand more or less irritant or poisonous chemicals which have been tested, relatively few produce cancer in the ordinary test animals of the laboratory. And when we tabulate those which are relatively highly active it is impossible to find any chemical character that is related to their cancer-producing power. In a book published in 1970, I made a suggestion that the only thing in common was that all the carcinogenic chemicals were non-biological in the sense that they were never part of the environment in which man and all his vertebrate ancestors evolved. They were substances for which enzymes to destroy them had not been developed. One can visualize small amounts of such substances entering the cell nucleus and, not being rapidly destroyed, some would persist long enough to do minor damage to part of the genetic mechanism, random damage that could produce any one of a thousand mutational changes. The damage must be in one sense quite trivial as the cell must by hypothesis still be capable of proliferation and of all the mutations that could be produced the only ones that could be recognized are the proliferative ones. Notice again how the random element predominates and how well it agrees with the fact that most of the drugs which can destroy cancer cells can also be shown to have cancer-producing capacity under other circumstances.

CANCER VIRUSES

In the last dozen years there has been a great concentration of research on the viruses which can produce cancer or leukaemia of mice, hamsters, and chickens. There is no doubt at all about the genuinely malignant character of the tumours which are produced but so far there is no convincing evidence that any human tumour is virus-induced. There is an important tumour affecting children in Central Africa (Burkitt lymphoma) which has a distribution strongly suggesting that in some way mosquitoes are concerned with its appearance. For some years the hypothesis was current that the tumours in these children were produced by a mosquito-borne virus perhaps of the group which contains the viruses of yellow fever or Japanese encephalitis. No such virus has been isolated and at the present time interest is swinging in another direction. The Burkitt lymphoma occurs only in heavily malarious areas: in Africa there is a striking similarity in the regional distribution of the two diseases. So in 1971 there is a growing opinion

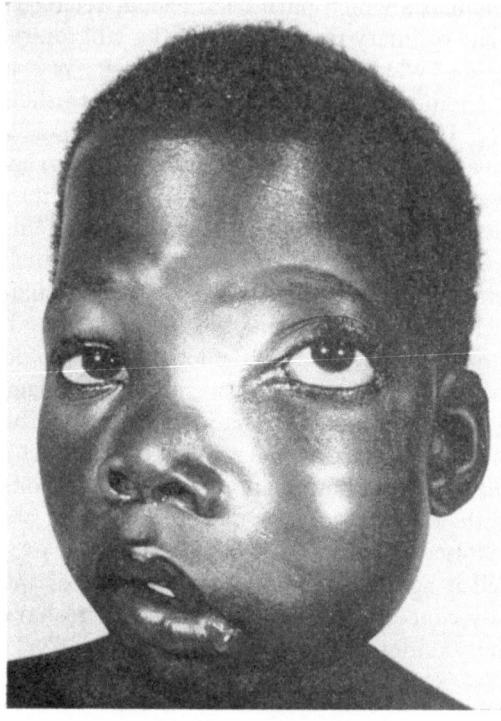

FIG. 37. Child with Burkitt lymphoma. (By courtesy of Mr D. P. Burkitt.)

that in some children the intense stimulation of the immune system by malarial infection results in the emergence of a malignant tumour (lymphoma) derived from one of the defence cells concerned. One must be definite, however, that despite ten years' intensive study neither the virus theory nor the malaria theory has established itself as any more than a speculation.

There may be almost a majority of younger cancer research men who think it likely that eventually cancer will be shown to be due to the action of 'slow viruses' which in the great majority of people persist without any visible effect. To me this is an unjustifiable and unscientific act of faith based on a failure to understand the significance of the work on viruses of laboratory animals.

I have often thought that an analysis of the basis of research on 'cancer viruses' would make an excellent introduction to population genetics and evolutionary theory. One incomplete but useful definition of life is 'the replication of organic pattern' with its implication that organic pattern whether of molecular structure, cell architecture or inborn behaviour can, once it appears, be made to apply to as large a population as can be developed by selective replication of the organism or unit concerned. Every one of the standard varieties of apple, Granny Smith, Jonathan, Delicious, and the rest, is derived each from a single seedling that has since been vegetatively propagated by grafting. Judging from the distribution of surnames amongst the Afrikaans-speaking people of South Africa, several of the original Dutch settlers of 1685 have now 12,500 or more direct descendants. There is no need to give other examples of the capacity of living things for exponential compound-interest growth wherever opportunity offers.

Let us now consider the situation in a cancer research laboratory where a good experimentalist is looking for a cancer virus of mice. He will presumably have a number of pure line strains of mice and if he detects a lump in a mouse over a year old he will be liable to examine the lump in detail and probably transfer fragments of its tissue to half a dozen mice of the same strain. If nothing happens the experiment ends forthwith but if a new generation of tumours is produced it continues. Soon a new line of transmissible cancer cells is available for study. In various ways, sublines, mutant derivatives of the original cell line, will be developed and propagated. Some of them will be more virulent multiplying more rapidly in new recipients than the original, some may be adapted to grow in different strains of mice. At intervals, tests are made to see whether an extract of the tumour freed from living cells can transmit the cancer. If he continues with sufficient perseverance the investigator may well find that perhaps in a proportion of baby mice some tumours are so produced. Efforts are now redoubled; each success provides material for further propagation, 'failures' are discarded. Eventually a full-blown cancer virus is to hand, yet it is highly probable that it has been derived from a virus which in the whole course of its evolutionary history was never associated with cancer until it entered that laboratory.

Since the development of modern methods of isolating and studying viruses in tissue culture, quite fantastically large numbers of differentiable types of virus have been isolated. Many are proven or potential agents of infectious disease but the number of what have been called 'viruses in search of a disease' is vastly greater. These are the viruses found unexpectedly in tissue cultures from apparently normal animals, isolated from mosquitoes or appearing when conventional studies of throat swabbings or faeces for disease-producers are made. They are genuine enough viruses but there is no evidence that they have been producing disease. In a rather similar fashion, whenever electron-micrographs of tissues from normal animals are closely scrutinized for 'virus-like particles' they are liable to be found even if parallel studies of the same tissues in attempts to isolate viruses have been fruitless. It is in fact quite clear that the smallest living units—biological purists nowadays will not allow us to call viruses organisms—are as diverse in form and function and occupy as wide a range of ecological niches as any group of organisms. In addition, as an ex-virologist once deeply interested in variation and adaptation in viruses like influenza, I have a real personal knowledge of how wide a range of mutants can be obtained from the descendants of a single virus unit.

All viruses must live at the expense of some living cell, from bacteria upwards to mammalian cells, but they do not necessarily damage cells in the process or, if they do, they may affect so small a proportion that no symptoms can be detected. These casual viruses are no more than nuisances to most virologists and very few of them have been sufficiently studied for anything to be known about their ecology, how any particular type manages to survive indefinitely in nature—what is its ecological niche. All that we can be certain of, is that in any population of laboratory mice—or of hamsters, monkeys, or men—one or more of a wide possible range of harmless or inconspicuously harmful viruses will be present in some of the tissues of some of the animals.

It is well known that viruses in general multiply more actively in rapidly proliferating embryonic or tumour cells—the types of cells used in most tissue cultures—and there are good biochemical reasons why this should be so. If an animal has developed a malignant tumour and at the same time is carrying a virus that can live quietly at the expense of the animal's normal cells it is likely also to be present in the tumour, as a rule in larger number than in any normal tissue.

We can now return to the laboratory in which the new cancer virus is to be discovered and consider the power of the selective evolutionary environment that is provided by an experimenter who is looking for a virus that will cause cancer. He knows what he is looking for, tumour cells which will grow readily on transfer to the next host animal, a virus that will be constantly associated with tumour cells and finally, a virus which will provoke malignant growth, initially in a newborn animal. He is dealing with two mutable entities, a tumour cell line and a virus species and he has a variety of techniques to favour any mutant moving in the right direction. He knows that he can build up large populations of desired mutants and will automatically discard any line of cell or virus which does not proliferate. It is not specially easy to persuade a virus to mutate to what is required of a cancer virus and there are only a half a dozen or so cancer viruses of mice which have been fully studied. Luck as well as perseverance is necessary. The basic requirements are:

1. That the virus should be able to multiply in the cell without killing it or seriously interfering with its capacity to multiply;

2. That in a proportion of infected cells, inheritable changes in the genetic mechanism of the cell should be induced. These may result from fragments of virus nucleic acid getting caught up with the cells DNA and randomly distorting its function in some direction or some other type of interference yet to be particularized;

3. That a proportion of the mutant cells so produced are cancer cells. If it is physically possible for a virus to produce by any mutation or sequence of mutations a descendant with these characters, the classic procedure will eventually result in its appearance and isolation.

There is only one established instance where it can be said with some justification that a virus produces cancer in nature. Domestic fowls are subject to infection with a group of 'leukoviruses' which are RNA viruses somewhat resembling the influenza viruses in their structure. In general the viruses do no visible harm but there is good evidence, though perhaps not real proof, that infection results in the appearance late in the life of the affected birds of a number of chronic pathological changes which would not occur in birds free of the virus. There may still be some confusion with the results of a different group of viruses but the current interpretation is that lesions consisting of accumulations of lymphocytes in various organs and, more rarely, proliferative conditions of the blood cells are due to the leukoviruses. More rarely still, solid tumours may be produced of which by far the best known is the famous Rous sarcoma. Viruses can usually be obtained from these rare malignant conditions which produce equivalent disorders in closely related birds but there is always a patchy irregularity in the results.

One can hardly consider twentieth-century poultry farming as providing a normal ecology for *Gallus bankiva* but, even so, the leukosis viruses seem to have established on the whole a satisfactory *modus vivendi* with their hosts. The commonest situation is for the virus to be transmitted by the egg and to produce a continuing latent infection without symptoms. With the large scale of the industry and the interest of specialist veterinary consultants, there is opportunity for mutant viruses to arise and for their effects to be recognized and investigated. In a real sense this allows the first stage of the process I described for the laboratory to take place in the poultry farm. Then in the laboratory the investigator can continue with the artificially intense selective process that is necessary for the emergence of an accepted cancer-producing (oncogenic) virus.

My great objection to the hypothesis that any human cancer is a direct result of virus infection is my inability to conceive of a selective process in nature that could be equivalent to the laboratory procedure. Considering the extreme rarity of cancer in wild animals I can see no way by which an ability to induce cancer could favour the survival of a virus species. Neither can I see anything in human biology which could have power to evolve human cancer viruses; except by deliberate human effort directed to such an end. One could perhaps produce a science-fiction tale of the psychopathic genius provided, through the connivance of some all-powerful Leader, with unlimited human embryos, tissue cultures, and babies for his experiments. What he would do with the human cancer virus when he produced it is beyond my imagination. But, short of such absurdities, I believe that we can forget about the possibility of any of the common forms of cancer being of virus origin.

But queer things have happened in the evolutionary history of life and it would be wise to leave some scope for pure random coincidence—that without any biological logic a virus surviving between water-birds and mosquitoes in Central Africa should, when babies are infected, give rise to the disfiguring jaw tumour that we call Burkitt lymphoma. Such a possibility can never be ruled out of consideration but so far none has been established.

MOLECULAR BIOLOGY AND CANCER

Any of the other aspects of cancer research that I have mentioned could provide opportunities for expansion and interpretation but I think it would fit best with the general approach of this book to look rather critically at that perennially repeated justification for work in molecular biology—that all competently done research in fundamental aspects of biology will help toward discovering the cause and cure of cancer. I believe that most scientists who make this claim, usually to justify public support for their own work, feel that they are virtually compelled by social forces to tell this white lie with as much apparent conviction as they can muster. They know that their own work is rated as good by their peers, who are concerned not at all with its bearing on cancer but deeply with its originality, its integrity of approach and interpretation, the elegance of the methods used, and the implications it will have for the interpretation of other biological phenomena. They are rightly proud of their achievement and equally rightly feel that they have won the right to go on with their researches. But their money comes from politicians, bankers, foundations who are not capable of recognizing the nature of the scientist's attitude to science and who still feel, as I felt myself thirty years ago, that medical research is concerned only in preventing or curing human disease. So our scientists say what is expected of them, their grants are renewed and both sides are uneasily aware that it has all been a basically dishonest piece of play-acting—but then most public functions are.

Most of the reasons for scepticism about the 'usefulness' of molecular biology have been given in Chapter 4. In essence there is only one reason, the impossible complexity of living structure and particularly of the informational machinery of the cell. When we come to look specifically at the possibility of finding the 'cause of cancer' through increasing knowledge of cytology and molecular biology, a little more can be said. The most optimistic approach would require the assumption that there is one specific deviation from normal biochemical function that makes a cell cancerous. This possibility is worth some consideration. In the first place whatever the change responsible it is inheritable in the cancer cell line, it is due to an informational change in the cells' nucleic acid. For reasons I have already discussed, deliberate manipulation of genetic material is out. Culling at the appropriate level is the only approach to genetic deviation or disaster. We must look for action at some more accessible level than the informational nucleic acid. Any single genetic change will be mediated by modification or deletion of some functional protein, change in which may have secondary results which by hypothesis lead to uncontrolled proliferation. If the nature of the change in the functional protein—presumably an enzyme—and the nexus between that change and the uncontrolled proliferation of the cell were known, how could that knowledge be utilized to cure a diagnosed cancer? There are two main possibilities: to supply something that is missing or to use the changed activity of the cancer cell to attract something which will destroy it. It would be unwise to eliminate possibilities that are as yet unthought of but, as things stand, the only hope for the first approach would be with rare 'hormone conditioned' tumours which immediately invalidates our original premise of a single common factor responsible for the cancerous state. The most optimistic dream for cancer treatment would probably be to find a drug which would block an enzyme (modified from some normal enzyme) which was responsible for malignant proliferation and was not present in normal cells. If blocking of the enzyme resulted in death of the cell, so much the better.

If cancer resulted from a uniform deviation of cell metabolism, one could reasonably hope for some means of biochemical attack. If, as everything suggests, cancers represent an almost infinitely heterogeneous group of abnormal cell lines whose only common feature is that they can engage in inadequately controlled proliferation, hope along these lines must vanish. It has been suggested that a semi-empirical approach would be possible even accepting the great diversity of cancers. This would involve removing the primary tumour surgically and establishing the cancer cells in tissue culture. Then, in much the same way as bacteria from a wound infection are tested for their sensitivity to different antibiotics, the tissue cultures could be tested against a wide selection of enzyme-blocking drugs. The results would, hopefully, allow the use of the most effective against any secondary cancer that might eventually appear. Research along these lines is already in progress but unless there is a completely new approach to the synthesis of appropriate drugs, its practical success is likely to be minimal. One major difficulty will be that secondary deposits of cancer nearly always represent more invasive mutant forms of the primary cancer cells.

CANCER IMMUNITY

Similar study of tissue cultures of the cells from a patient's primary cancer is also being done in an attempt to apply the principles of immunity to a wide diversity of tumours. In the next chapter we shall be concerned with the implications of immunity for what we can call the natural history of cancer. But it will be convenient to introduce the topic here in so far as it is potentially relevant to the treatment of cancer.

It has been known for centuries that very, very rarely a typical cancer will 'miraculously' wither away leaving only a puckered scar. Nowadays such disappearance of an untreated cancer is rarer still but we do have significant numbers of cases where a surgeon has carried out a palliative operation or merely convinced himself that the condition was quite inoperable and the patient has recovered. This is the most dramatic evidence for the modern conviction that the body can mount a resistance against cancer that can sometimes be successful even against advanced disease. That resistance is immunological and depends on the fact that most, perhaps all, cancer cells have surfaces which can be recognized as abnormal, as being different from any of the cells functioning normally in the body.

Modern immunology is for many of us the most fascinating area of current biological research. I have been in the thick of it for many years and have written extensively about both general aspects and the applications of immunology to cancer. Immunology is immensely wide-ranging and its theoretical basis is by no means simple. In Chapter 1, I outlined the two distinctive types of immunological response to foreign material in the body. Once foreignness has been recognized, appropriate cells, capable of reacting with the foreign chemical patterns, multiply and mount two distinct types of attack. The first group of cells are responsible for 'cell-mediated immunity' and they are specially important in dealing with foreign cells whether these are grafted from someone else or arise as cancer from normal cells. The second group of immune cells are 'plasma cells' which produce antibody, a soluble protein—a whole series of proteins really—which by combining with foreign cell, micro-organism, or protein can facilitate its rapid removal from the body.

Both types of cell populations develop to some extent against all foreign patterns but cell-mediated immunity is by far the most important where attack on cancerous or grafted cells is concerned. With some over-simplification, one can say that when the attacking immune cells come into contact with the foreign 'target' cells, an almost explosive interaction occurs which damages both cells and leads directly or indirectly to the destruction of the foreign cells. Antibody which will also react with the foreign target cells is usually formed but has little effect as a rule.

One of the important results of working with pure line animals amongst which a cancer can be freely transferred was that it allowed the recognition that tumours could be shown capable of provoking an immune reaction. Here is an account of an experiment which had very important implications. As always, it is a simplified account but it presents the essentials of an experiment done in Klein's laboratory in Stockholm around 1956. A cancer-producing chemical, MCA, was injected into the leg muscles of a dozen mice of a single pure line X, tumours developed in the muscles and, under anaesthesia, the leg involved was amputated and the tumour cells from each of six such tumours grown separately in tissue culture. When adequate supplies of tumour cells had been grown some were partially killed with X-rays to make something equivalent to a vaccine. Klein then took six groups of the same pure line mice and vaccinated them, one group with tumour A, the next with tumour B, and so on. In due course he tested mice of each group with living cancer cells of A, B, C, D, E, and F tumours. The result was a clear-cut one, mice vaccinated with A together with the original, now three-legged mouse within which tumour A had developed, were immune against tumour A. No tumours developed in them but A cells could produce tumours as readily in mice vaccinated with B, C, D, etc., as in normal mice. A immunized only against A, B against B, and so on.

This was a rather special experiment, not all experiments of that general type give such clear-cut results but the basic findings hold, that tumours produced by chemicals provoke immunity that is

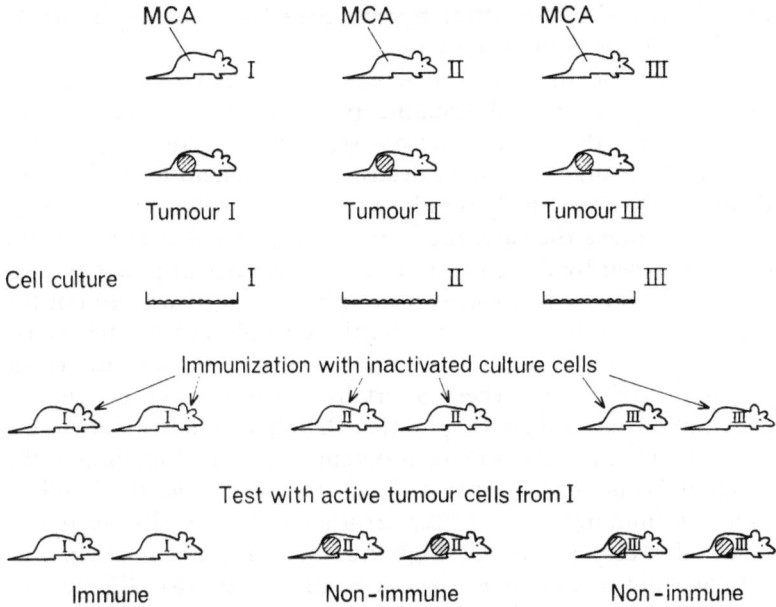

F IG. 38. Klein's experiment with pure line mice injected with the carcinogen MCA. Each tumour immunizes only against itself.

almost wholly limited to their own type of tumour. Each tumour has, as we say, its own individual antigenic specificity. The other thing to be noted is that this immunity requires special artifices to bring it to light. If the original mice had not had their tumours removed surgically they would all eventually have died of cancer. Today many people hope that we may be able to apply immune processes to the treatment of cancer but if we look at that experiment closely we can see most of the difficulties.

First, all tumours are individual. One cannot use one man's cancer cells to immunize another man against his, and until a cancer has actually developed there is nothing, immunologically speaking, that can be done. *Second*, a developing cancer that has reached the level at which it can be diagnosed has almost by definition overcome any spontaneous immune response. Only after most of it has been removed, is the immune paralysis it induced likely to disappear. *Third*, once a tumour has developed, cells within its mass are liable to further mutation which may render them more resistant to attack by immune cells or change the whole quality of their immune pattern.

Probably the most that one can legitimately say about the practical significance of immune processes in the treatment of cancer is that they may be necessary, as it were, to complete the job. If, after surgery or other destructive treatment by anti-cancer drugs or X-rays, small numbers of cancer cells remain, as is probably always the case, the immune response first induced and then paralysed by the growing tumour, may regain power to deal with them. There is a widespread opinion that, if it were not for the body's own immune response, there would be very few satisfactory results of cancer treatment. One notices, too, in recent discussions of cancer surgery, a certain distrust of too wide removal of lymph glands which, despite their liability to be sites of secondary tumours, are also the main potential source of immune cells.

There is one final point that should be made about the implications of immunity for cancer treatment. I have already mentioned the disconcertingly high number of cancers arising in patients given immunosuppressive drugs (p. 18). These are essentially cytotoxic drugs acting to some extent on all actively proliferating cells and some of them have been used for the chemotherapy of leukaemia. Conversely, any drug that has potentialities for selective killing of malignant cells is almost automatically immunosuppressive to some degree. In theory at least, chemotherapy of cancer could be a two-edged weapon. Conceivably the degree of destruction of malignant cells might be of less significance than the depression of any power to react immunologically against surviving cancer cells. It may be that this is one of the reasons why the chemotherapy of cancer has never become a standard method of treatment.

8

IMMUNOLOGICAL SURVEILLANCE
AND AGEING

All men are mortal and nowadays an increasing proportion are being given the opportunity to die a natural death, which could be defined as one which is preceded and eventually provoked by the increasing vulnerability of old age. Everyone resents old age to some degree and the myth of an elixir of youth has been extant for centuries. Every advance in medicine and biology in the last hundred years has been scrutinized for its bearing on the understanding of senescence and the amelioration of the indignities of old age. In the field of microbiology and immunology, Metchnikoff was preaching the virtues of changing the bacterial flora of the large bowel in the 1890s and the most recent discussion of genetic and immunological aspects of ageing is probably in a paper of mine published in August 1970.

The first stage of our discussion must be to characterize those features of old age in man (and to some extent in other mammals) which offer leads to an understanding of the essential biological processes involved.

CHARACTERISTICS OF THE AGEING PROCESS

I have mentioned vulnerability as a major aspect of ageing, using the word in the sense that any type of damaging impact from the environment will have a greater liability to 'cause serious bodily harm' or to kill than it would have on a younger person. An elderly woman will fracture the neck of her femur with a fall that would have seemed trivial to her twenty years earlier. When a 'new' infectious disease affects a population with no past immunity the mortality rises characteristically with age. This holds also for what we tend to call nonspecific respiratory infections shown on the death certificate as 'bronchitis', 'influenza', or 'bronchopneumonia', in which a variety of viruses and bacteria may be concerned.

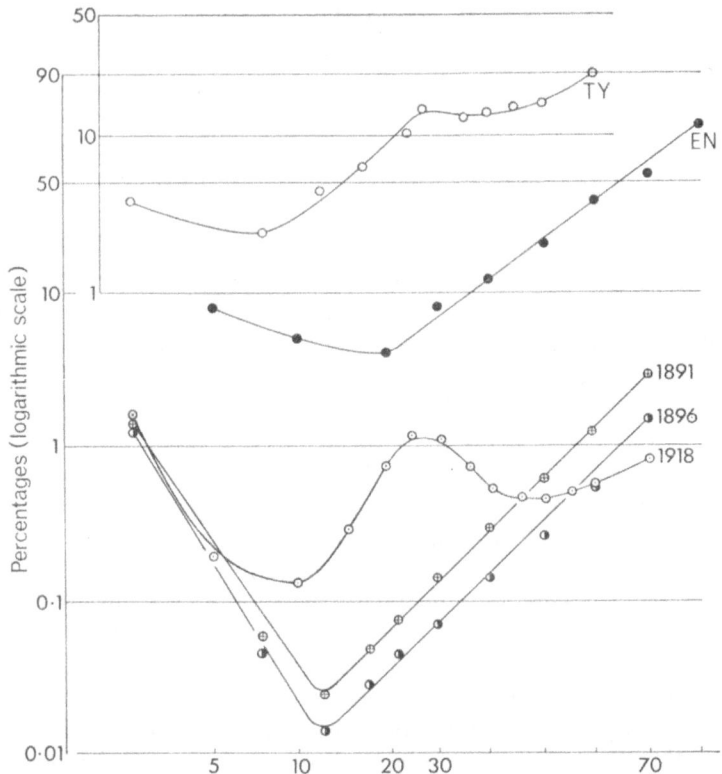

FIG. 39. To show increased mortality with age from (*a*) specific conditions to which the individuals are non-immune: the example shows fatality rates for typhoid fever, Western Australia (TY) and St Louis encephalitis (EN) (1933). The typhoid scale is inset. (*b*) Infections of a non-specific character: the example shows infections in two 'influenza' years (1891 and 1918) and a 'non-influenza' year (1896). (Note. The time-scale changes from logarithmic to linear at twenty-five years.)

As will be seen in the examples shown in Fig. 39 this rising vulnerability to infectious disease is one of the most clearly documented aspects of ageing. It is the first intimation of something which will become a central feature of this discussion, the progressive weakening and ineffectiveness of immune responses with old age.

The conventional image of a very old person is of someone frail, bowed, and small with thin heavily wrinkled skin. Those physical

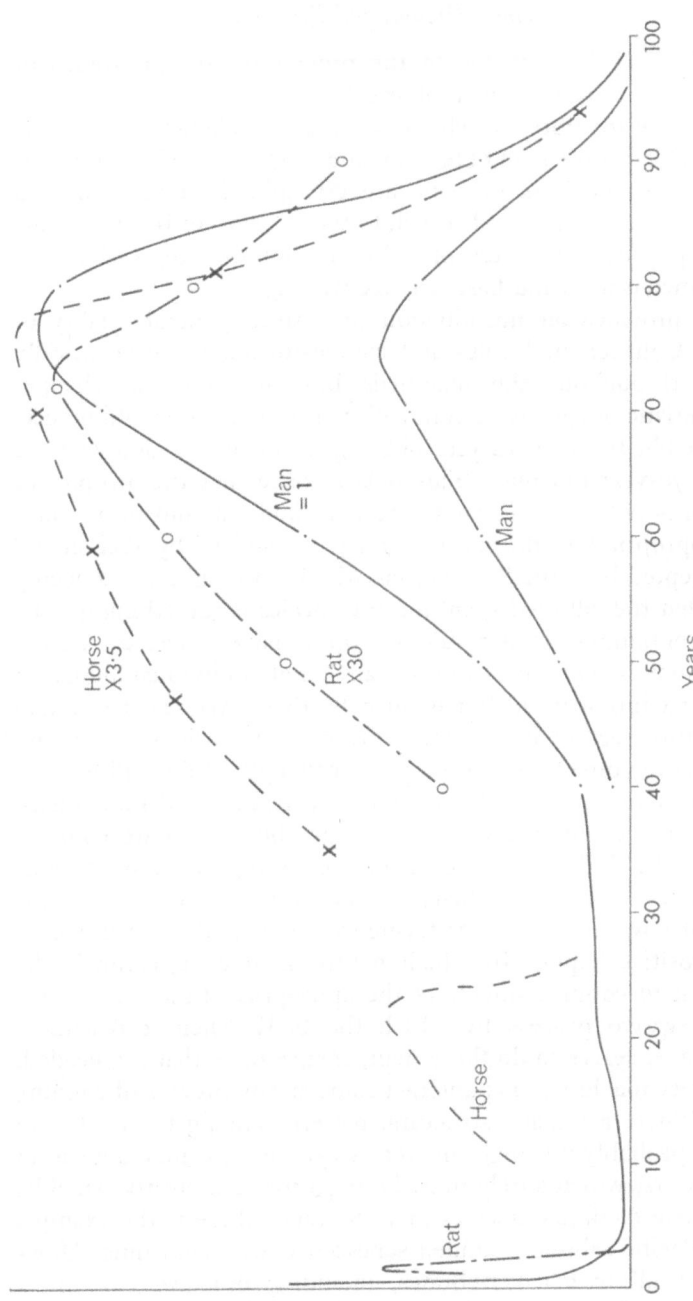

FIG. 40. Programmed ageing. The distribution of deaths by ages for rat, horse, and man, showing peaks of mortality at 22 months, 22 years, and 76 years, respectively. Also in the upper series of curves, with time-scales adjusted in the sequence 30 times, 3·5 times, and unaltered to show general resemblance of curves of natural death as a function of life-span.

findings are primarily due to the progressive disappearance of collagen, so is the fragility of the bones. Collagen is the most important of the fibres which give form and resilience to the body, it is the chief component of tendons and ligaments, and the minerals which form the bulk of bone are crystallized in relation to a collagen matrix which adds much to the strength of bone. Change in the physical character of collagen and its progressive disappearance is a second basic change with age.

This provides an introduction to a third general quality of ageing. Collagen molecules and composite fibres are chemically similar throughout the mammals but the chemical changes characteristic of age are seen in collagen from a 2-year-old mouse, a 3-year-old rat, or a 12-year-old dog in much the same state as from a 70-year-old man. This tells at once that the atrophy of collagen is not a simple matter of wear and tear but occurs at a time appropriate to the species. It was recognized by Weissmann and accepted by virtually everyone who has thought about ageing since, that the 'allotted span' for any species is something genetically programmed as a result of evolutionary processes. In the wild it may be extremely rare for any single individual animal to reach that inbuilt span but it must be there. We can be certain that nature sees to it that for a given species the number and timing of the offspring and the standard length of life will be such as to maintain an optimal density and distribution of individuals. That makes evolutionary common sense but, when we come to look at the individual organism, we recognize some serious problems. That the individual grows old and dies, is the inescapable fact, but how are we to start trying to understand it? Does something positive happen by which nature, as it were, compels the organism to commit suicide at the appropriate time? Or, is it a more negative process by which the body when it reaches a critical age, ceases to do those maintenance tasks that are needed, as in every machine, to counteract some steady process of running down? There are many structural patterns amongst animals and there is probably no single answer. Mayfly imagos may die within a few hours, which surely must be regarded as a positive suicide. Even if we confine ourselves to vertebrates, there is the example of the Pacific salmon's sudden senescence after spawning. However, for all higher vertebrates, including ourselves, we must probably look for the second type of situation, a fading-out of maintenance, a sort of built-in obsolescence. There are various semi-technical ways of expressing it, that nature loses interest after age x, that potentially lethal genetic characters have their expression delayed until after age x, but they tell us little or nothing of the nature of the biological clock that determines x.

So far, we have been concerned with negative factors in ageing, vulnerability with loss of effective immune responses, loss of elasticity, and atrophy of collagen. There are also positive disadvantages of old age in the sense that many diseases are so characteristically confined, by and large, to old age that they either form part of the picture of senescence or are very closely related to the basic processes of ageing. These diseases include cancer, a range of auto-immune diseases, and another range of conditions associated with degenerative changes in blood vessels of which coronary disease (heart attacks) and 'cerebral vascular accidents' (strokes) are the most conspicuous.

The role of the thymus

In outlining the importance of immunology for the understanding of modern medicine in Chapter 1, I indicated that much of my interest was in the possibility that immune responses might play a significant part in the natural history of cancer. I gave an outline of the two systems of immune cells, the B-cells which produce antibody and the T-cells (thymus-dependent cells) which are responsible for cell-mediated immunity, which means simply that the immune cells are themselves responsible for damage done to the target cells against which the immune attack is directed.

Of these two systems the B system which is responsible for production of antibody is of relatively little significance in relation to old age and cancer. I shall pay much more attention to the thymus-dependent (T) system and I shall go into considerably more detail about that still rather mysterious organ, the thymus, before trying to give an outline of its function in immunity.

All young mammals are born with a large thymus, so-called because of a resemblance of its shape to that of two slightly overlapping leaves of thyme. It lies behind the breast-bone and over the great vessels of the heart and is made up mostly of lymphocytes. These are ubiquitous cells just as characteristic of spleen and lymph glands as of the thymus and widely distributed elsewhere in the body. Modern dogma makes the lymphocyte the primary cell concerned with immunity. New lymphocytes are produced in the three sets of organs I have mentioned and probably also in the bone marrow. There is a constant circulation, cells from the thymus, spleen, and bone marrow entering the blood directly, while those from all the lymph glands of the body pass into lymph channels that collect into two lymphatic trunks. These open into the great veins just before they enter the heart. Lymphocytes are constantly leaving the circulation and in the course of their various activities are destroyed in large numbers. Over-all the number in the blood remains nearly constant.

Present teaching has it that the T–D lymphocytes have become differentiated for their particular immune function while they were developing in the thymus from ancestral cells which came from the bone marrow. The production of these T–D immunocytes, or defence cells, reaches its maximum very soon after birth when the thymus itself has its greatest size relative to the body as a whole. In man the absolute maximum size is reached at the age of 10 or 12 years. Then it diminishes in size and becomes functionally insignificant in middle age. Most individuals over 60 have only two small fatty lobes with some fibrous tissue to show where their thymuses used to be. This does not mean that there are no T–D immunocytes in the circulation and lymph tissues of an elderly individual. There are still many descendants of cells that were differentiated in the thymus but no *new* lines are being produced. Much more could be said about the T–D immune system but the important thing from our present point of view is that it is the system concerned with recognizing and dealing with foreign *cells*, either cells from another individual that have entered the body by grafting or injection, or cells which by somatic mutation have developed a new antigenic character. Recognition and response are functions of the immunocytes themselves and require cell surface to cell surface contact with the (foreign) target cell. Destruction of the target cell resulting in rejection of a skin graft or elimination of a cancer focus is a complex process initiated by the liberation of damaging drug-like agents by the cells in contact. These may result in death of both target cell and immunocyte and the activation of other normally inactive lymphocytes in the vicinity to add to the damaging effect.

Immunological surveillance

Over the last five years I have been writing a good deal about 'immunological surveillance' which is the concept that one of the biologically important reasons for the existence of an immune system is to deal with incipient malignant disease, with cancer. The T–D system, on my reading, is primarily there to recognize any little nidus of abnormal cells and nip it in the bud before it becomes too large and invasive to be dealt with. It is a surveillance function perpetually patrolling the body, as it were, for evildoers. The body and its immunocytes tolerate any normal chemical patterns that have a genetic right to be in the body. It is only when some unusual chemical configuration develops as a result of somatic mutation that T–D immunocytes are called into action— and we must remember that somatic mutation is constantly occurring.

The experimental evidence for the existence of immunological surveillance comes wholly from work with cancer induced in mice, rats, hamsters, and guinea-pigs, either by carcinogenic chemicals like MCA or the cancer viruses polyoma and SV 40. It is only an assumption that other mutations not potentially cancerous also develop antigens which could make them subject to surveillance.

Polyoma virus has already been mentioned as a possible agent to ferry a synthetic gene from the test-tube to the cells that need it for their rehabilitation. Its behaviour in mice or hamsters offers a particularly clear picture of immunological surveillance in action. In discussing cancer viruses it was mentioned that polyoma virus injected into an animal more than a week or two old had no effect apart from producing a minor immune response. In newborn mice or hamsters, injection of the virus gave rise with almost complete regularity to multiple tumours. This phenomenon has been analysed in depth and the current interpretation in brief is as follows: A proportion of infected cells are modified, 'transformed', so that they develop a new cell surface antigen TSTA (tumour specific transplantation antigen) different from any normal cell antigen of the animal but similar for all cells transformed by

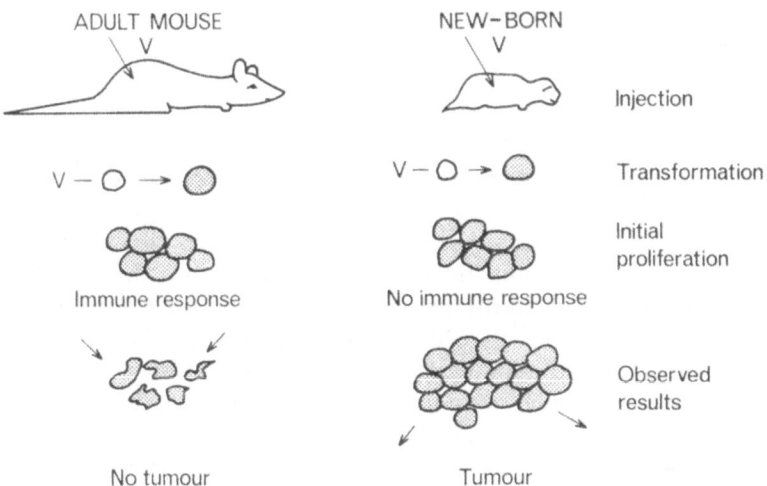

FIG. 41. To illustrate the results of injecting polyoma virus into adult and newborn mice. The absence of an immune response against the antigen on virus-transformed cells in the newborn animal allows the development of tumour. Where an immune response is possible in the adult the cells of the incipient tumour are destroyed.

polyoma virus. This happens in both newborn and adult mice. In the newborn some or all of the transformed cells proliferate to produce tumours, liberate TSTA, and paralyse the immune response. In the adult an immune response is called into action rapidly and any incipient tumours are dealt with by T-type immune cells and no tumours develop.

It may be of interest to mention a few of the experiments which have helped to establish this interpretation of what happens with polyoma virus and the more general concept of immunological surveillance.

Once a tumour has developed, the malignant cells can be transferred to an adult mouse of the same pure strain and produce a typical tumour. With transplantation the virus disappears and the tumour reveals its origin only by the TSTA it carries—some other differences are not relevant in the present context. Such a transplantable virus-free tumour is not, however, transplantable to a mouse of the right strain which has been immunized with live polyoma virus. This resistance shows that in the adult mouse, injection of virus has in fact produced tumour cells and TSTA and that the TSTA has immunized the mouse against both the initiated tumour cells and the subsequent test transplant.

There are three ways to produce a mouse with greatly diminished immunological capacity, one is to remove its thymus on the first day of life, the second is to give it an immunosuppressive drug and the third is to give it an anti-lymphocyte serum made against mouse lymphocytes in a rabbit. In grown mice treated in any of those ways, injection of polyoma virus will produce tumours.

Finally, in the opposite direction this time, there is one strain of mice, C57Bl, which is well known for its effective immune response against a variety of antigens. Baby mice of this strain do not produce tumours when inoculated with polyoma virus. This resistance could, in principle, be due to genetic inability of the strain to allow tumour growth or it could be due to an unusually early mobilization of an immune response against the first tumour cells produced. The choice between the two alternatives can be made by using the virus to induce tumour cells in a situation where there is no possibility of an immune response, i.e., in a tissue culture of C57Bl cells. Transformed cells from such a culture when injected in large enough number into grown mice produce typical transplantable polyoma tumours. The interpretation is clearly that immunological surveillance develops earlier in the C57Bl mouse than in other types.

A basically similar account could be given of the experiments which show that carcinogenic chemicals can also provoke tumours with new immune patterns, new TSTA's. Although there are some important differences the results point almost as clearly as those with polyoma virus to the importance of immunological surveillance. They bring out an additional point that has an important bearing on clinical matters.

Several of the substances which can produce cancer when painted on the skin or injected into the muscles of a mouse have what is called an immunosuppressive action which damps down or suppresses completely all types of immune response. Most people must have come across the term, immunosuppression, when reading about kidney and heart transplants. Such operations are only made possible by the use of immunosuppressive drugs which prevent the normal immune attack of the body on the foreign graft. The present view is that the immunosuppressive action of the chemical carcinogens used on mice probably plays a significant part in their cancer-producing effect. By neutralizing the surveillance function it prevents the body from rejecting any little focus of cancer that has begun to develop in the mouse.

This sort of thing does not happen only in the experimental cancer laboratory. As I have mentioned earlier, more than thirty cases of cancer have been reported as arising in patients who had been under long-continued treatment with immunosuppressive drugs after transplant operations. Statistically such cancers are many times more numerous than they would be in persons of similar ages not receiving such drugs. At the human level this unfortunate side-effect of kidney transplantation is probably the most decisive evidence of the surveillance role of the immune system in man.

Surveillance cannot, however, be wholly confined to malignant cells. If some particular type of common mutation eventually produces a large population of cells with the same altered surface but no tendency to proliferate unduly, then sooner or later these, too, are likely to be recognized and will provoke the appearance of T–D immunocytes that can interact with them. For fairly obvious reasons it will never be easy to establish the extent of somatic mutations which do not manifest themselves by proliferative advantage. Some deductions from general principles will therefore be necessary. We can reasonably assume that mutation must be at least as frequent in a somatic cell as in a germ cell and there is cogent evidence that mutation can occur while a cell is quiescent as well as when it is dividing. Once the fertilized ovum has begun to divide, any of its descendant cells may be subject to somatic mutation. Once a mutation has occurred and the cell concerned remains viable, that cell line will carry it indefinitely. Descendant cells within the line will also, of course, be potentially subject to further mutations. In other words the embryo starts with a clean slate but with every cell generation some mutations will occur and as the animal matures and ages, a progressively increasing number of cells will have undergone one, two, or more mutations. Toward the end of life it is probable that some of the more common types of somatic mutation are represented in a majority of cells. Several writers, notably Curtis, have felt that ageing may largely be the result of simple accumulation of somatic mutations. Others including Walford and myself while agreeing that this is important, feel that the characteristic stigmata of old age result much more from immunological responses and anomalies associated with somatic mutation.

Auto-immune disease

There is one further aspect of somatic mutation which is specially important because it involves the immunocytes themselves. Much has been written on the theme of immunological tolerance but only one point about it need be made here. An immunocyte must not, for obvious reasons, attack normal body cells—they are sacrosanct, tolerated by the whole immune system. No antibody production, no immune response must be made against anything which is rightfully present in the body.

But, even in nature, even in the living body, laws are not always obeyed. Wherever cells are multiplying there is a possibility of error in copying—of somatic mutation and when we are dealing with the immunocytes (defence cells) there is an important way in which certain mutations can change their character almost literally from good to evil. They may be changed so that they, as it were, mistakenly regard some normal type of cell as alien and to be attacked as a foreign cell would be. This attack, when it produces symptoms, represents auto-immune disease. But auto-immune mutant cells are basically like cancer cells, with an important difference. They multiply because they are stimulated to do so by contact with some normal body substance with which they can react. A normal immunocyte is made to proliferate by contact with the bacterial antigen that corresponds to its special character and when the bacterial infection is overcome, the immunocyte line shrinks almost to its normal insignificant population. But, if the stimulating antigen is a normal body component *always* present, the mutant immunocyte line behaves like a cancer under this constant stimulation. This is one of the standard ways cells can go wrong and almost certainly the body has several lines of defence against such auto-immune cells. Once cancer is diagnosed, its natural cure is very, very rare, but there are many, perhaps most, auto-immune diseases which show remissions and sometimes burn themselves out. For a number of reasons, none very convincing alone, but adding up to something significant, I believe that the most important final line of defence is the same as that against cancer cells, immunological surveillance.

AN IMMUNOLOGICAL HYPOTHESIS OF AGEING

At this stage I should warn the reader that I am unashamedly presenting an hypothesis about the nature of ageing which I helped to develop and about which I have been writing recently at a technical level. Under those circumstances I shall be biased in deciding that most of the alternative hypotheses are so improbable that it would only confuse matters to discuss them!

The essence of the approach that I shall use is that ageing is to a very large extent due to the exhaustion of the thymus-dependent system and probably also of the broader system of generalized circulating cells of which the T–D system is a specialized part. For the time being, we can set aside the obvious next question of why the immune system fades away with age. There are many good lines of evidence, some already mentioned, that all immune responses become less effective with age, and immunological surveillance will go the same way. On the other hand all effects of somatic mutation that are not lethal to cells go on accumulating. Back-mutation to normal can be forgotten for the simple reason that if the chance of any single point-mutation is one in a million, then the chance that a cell or a cell-line will both mutate and back-mutate at the same point, is one in a million millions. Mutant cells will go on developing further mutations and, if any such 'sequential' mutations give a proliferative advantage, the cell line will be so much further on the way toward malignancy. The concentration of cancer toward old age therefore has two main conditioning factors—the accumulation of somatic mutations by the simple elapse of time and the waning effect of immunological surveillance in nipping incipient cancer in the bud.

What I have said about the nature of auto-immune disease would necessarily imply that, like cancer, such auto-immune conditions will become more frequent in old age for the same reasons. If we allow for the fact, still not fully explained, that there are genetic differences in predisposition to auto-immune disease, the facts in regard to age incidence agree with this deduction.

The various forms of cancer and auto-immune disease are

important amongst the diseases of old age but vascular accidents due to degeneration of arteries with either blocking or bursting to give the acute symptoms that we call heart attacks or strokes, are more important. In addition there are even larger numbers of persons who become senile with a variety of bodily weaknesses rather than specific disease and who die by almost random mishaps when their vulnerability reaches the danger point. We know that these degenerations have a genetic element in their causation, in part concerned with how they handle cholesterol in the body. Environmental factors—cigarette smoking, over-eating with overweight as its indicator, excessive consumption of alcohol, social worries, and personal disasters—all these have been incriminated and figures given in support. There remains the third universe of significance, somatic mutation and immunological reactions to changed cells.

By the time old age is reached, many types of mutant cells *not* on the road to malignancy will be scattered through the tissues and there will be enough of some types to allow an immune response against them. This is a deduction which it may be impossible to prove or disprove, either at the clinical or experimental level. If it occurs it will be a slowly progressive process. One might picture mutant X being common in the cells lining the blood vessels, the vascular endothelium. Once an immune response had produced a significant number of anti-X immunocytes, we should find gradually increasing numbers of episodes in which an X cell or a group of them are being 'attacked' by anti-X immunocytes. In each episode a little focus of damage also involving adjacent cells will be produced with trivial effects in itself but in the long run contributing to a degeneration of the vascular system. There are hints that this does occur but nothing approaching proof.

Similar types of damage to *normal* tissue cells in blood vessels or elsewhere could be produced by auto-immune processes. When, with age, the efficiency of immunological surveillance is waning and active families of auto-immune cells are able to flourish, chronic organ damage of some sort is to be expected.

The essence of the argument is that a progressive run down of immune surveillance with age could be the dominating factor to account for the association of cancer, auto-immune disease, and degenerative changes with ageing. Genetic and environmental factors are not thereby excluded.

We are left with the question of why the immune responses run down and with the need to justify the assumption that the loss of effectiveness of the immune system precedes and in a real sense is responsible for degeneration and loss of effectiveness in other parts of the body. The loss of effectiveness of all immune reactions with age is well established but we have not accounted for that weakening nor have we brought into the picture another major feature of ageing referred to earlier, the degeneration and partial disappearance of collagen. Another aspect of age, too, must be introduced at this stage. The modern view is that the organs primarily concerned with immunity are the lymphoid tissues, spleen, lymph glands, thymus, and, in part, bone marrow. All these lymphoid tissues shrink with age, spleen and lymph nodes moderately, but the thymus at an altogether more rapid rate. There is no functional thymus at all in old age and very little after 40 or 50.

As the T–D cells are those which are responsible for surveillance, one naturally looks for some relationship between the virtual disappearance of the thymus in middle life and thereafter the steady rise in cancer and auto-immune disease. One must not be too unsophisticated in making such a deduction, the thymus-dependent system is much more than the thymus. Taking everything into consideration I am inclined to believe that it is the atrophy of the T–D system that, primarily through the consequent failure of immunological surveillance, determines when senescence will occur. In one sense the biological clock can be located in the thymus and its dependent cells. When they fade away, 'maintenance' ceases and all the evils of old age are set loose.

The Hayflick limit

But we cannot stop there. Once again we have to go deeper and look for possible reasons why thymus and T–D system atrophy around 1 year in mice and around 40 years in man. This brings us to the Hayflick limit and, once we reach that, we have gone about as deep as we can go. Hayflick is a tissue-culture man working at the Wistar Institute in Philadelphia. He found, and others have confirmed, that if he started a tissue culture line from human embryonic cells these cells would, under the best conditions, multiply for about fifty generations. Then they died unless somewhere along the line there had been a mutation to a more or less cancerous state.

Apparently there is a limit of ± 50 to the number of times an embryonic human cell can go on dividing as a somatic cell. Hayflick would probably say that if we went back to the starting cell, the fertilized ovum, perhaps another 20 generations would have to be added. For all somatic cells, only those $20 + 50$ generations are possible. However, if you do the sums and work out how many cells are produced when you multiply by 2, 70 successive times you will have ample numbers of cells to populate that four-dimensional clone which is one way of looking at the life of a man. The number is 10^{21}. All this refers only to somatic cells. The germ cells must have other rules.

One can only guess that there is some metabolic requirement at work. To the best of my knowledge there are no more detailed suggestions and the technical requirements of the experiments and the fact that '50' means something between 38 and 64, have made it difficult to extend the story to other species. Hayflick feels strongly that the phenomenon is basic to ageing, and I find the idea very attractive—though I am prepared to change my mind if new evidence calls for that. There are gerontologists who are quite unconvinced that the Hayflick limit is any more than an artificial laboratory phenomenon due to some unrecognized weakness in tissue culture technique. Its attraction may well be simply because it allows a self-consistent theory of ageing to be formulated which covers most of the facts and has not yet been disproved. It takes more or less the following form: Each species has a basic inbuilt biological clock in the form of an appropriate Hayflick limit to the number of divisions in somatic cells. Once any line reaches the limit appropriate to its species the cells can go no further, there can be no more descendants and the tissue which should receive them must atrophy. It follows that if a certain set of cell lines vital to continued life exhaust their quota of generations more rapidly than any others, the signs of old age will be the changes which result from the absence of these particular cells. We know that the most active turnover of relevant cells is in those lines which lead to thymus-dependent lymphocytes and we deduce that the stem cells which give rise to collagen-synthesizing fibroblasts also exhaust their quota early. The plasma cell series of immunocytes may represent another set of lines which is liable to run out of steam at about the same ages. Everywhere in such discussions as this, one comes up against the extreme difficulty of tracing the movement and lineages of the cells we are interested in. Most of those who have investigated these matters but by no means all, would agree that there was a good case for the unitary theory of the origin of the circulating cells. This holds that a line of almost wholly undifferentiated stem cells is maintained in the bone marrow from which the various blood cells and other cells concerned with maintenance and repair, as contrasted with the specialized functional cells of organs, are derived. If lymphocytes of the T–D system, the collagen-producing fibroblasts in every tissue of the body and the plasma cell system which produces antibody, are all part of the same stem cell system, it would be reasonable that they should all tend to reach Hayflick limits around the same time and before the rest of the body is affected. It may be that this immunological theory of ageing is a little too slick, that we are looking at only one facet of a very complex matter. But, as the matter stands today, it seems to be the best general statement we can find.

There are other approaches to ageing than the combination of somatic mutation and immunological response that I have favoured and which, in a slightly different form, is supported by Walford in his book, *The Immunological Theory of Aging*. None of them has been quite so fully developed, but an indication for the need to keep an open mind can be given by mentioning two experimental findings that do not show any obvious relationship to the immunological theory. Since they represent the only examples of experimentally *increased* longevity, they must be given due weight:

1. If immediately on weaning, rats are given a diet inadequate in calories but balanced in regard to protein and vitamins, development of sexual maturity can be delayed for nearly three years. If they are then given a full diet they may survive for a total of five years, which is much longer than rats survive on normal laboratory diet. There are obviously interesting things to be learnt about thymus sizes and cellular turnover in these rats if they are to fit into the picture.

2. In industry, if one wishes to improve the 'longevity' of rubber tyres or keep fats from going rancid, one adds anti-oxidants, organic chemicals which inhibit oxidation processes. It is claimed

that with proper dosage of some anti-oxidants such as mercapto-
ethylamine, mice live longer than their untreated litter mates
under the same basic conditions. It may be that there is a clue
here to the nature of the Hayflick limit—or in ten years' time the
finding may be seen as the beginning of some entirely different
approach.

CAN HUMAN LIFE BE PROLONGED?

At the clinical level there have been ideas that age comes on as
sex hormone levels fall, since the days of Voronoff and Steinach.
Modern views are more sophisticated and most activities are in
the gynaecological field. Several groups are interested in showing
that post-menopausal women treated with a proper balance of
hormones are less liable to weakening of the bones and to cancer
of the uterine cervix as well as being generally healthier. No one,
so far, however, has been able to satisfy the critically minded that
his results prove his case.

Many opinions have been expressed as to what will lengthen
life or what will shorten it. In the play that Bernard Shaw wrote
on the topic *Back to Methuselah*, his contemporary prime minister
asks the brothers Barnabas whether their elixir is sour milk or
lemons or something else. Of suggestions I have come across in
my reading the one that interests me most is that there may be
length of life to be gained by winning success and recognition in
professions sheltered from social stress. An American sociologist
took a properly chosen sample of men whose biographies were
included in the American *Who's Who* for 1950 and followed the
mortality amongst them for the next twelve years. Making the
appropriate actuarial adjustments to give a single figure for the
mortality of each professional group he found that American
scientists well known enough to be entered in the book had a death-
rate 79 per cent of that for the whole *Who's Who* group covering
the professions, politicians, businessmen, and all the rest. This was
one of the lowest values, while journalists were the highest, with
210 per cent of the average mortality. There are available general
US figures for mortality in occupational groups including the
professions. Comparison of scientists in *Who's Who* with the
general group of scientists of the same age showed that the former
had only 32 per cent of the mortality of unselected scientists.

It may be that academic scientists of repute have a sheltered life, but to say that has the implication that worry and disappointment shorten life and calls for some explanation at the physiological level. There is the same implication and question in a recent study of 270 men, 60–94 years old, which found that 'work satisfaction and morale' are better predictors of longevity than physical fitness, smoking history, nutritional status, or parents' age at death.

Even if we knew much more about ageing it would not necessarily give us a practical means of extending the average life span. Nature is not going to co-operate with us in keeping men or any other animal alive for much beyond the span she has allotted. What I think may be a useful approach to prolonging the period of *healthy* old age is, however, suggested by one characteristic of the thymus. Every serious illness, whether an infection, an injury, or anything else requiring hospitalization, causes rapid atrophy of the functional part of the thymus. If we agree with the view I have adopted, we could claim that each episode uses up part of the quota of thymus-dependent cells and by hypothesis shortens life. Anything we can do to provide a childhood and early life free from illness is in itself likely to favour freedom from untimely illness in old age. That, I think, runs so well with traditional wisdom and also with statistics of mortality that it is both sound advice and, I like to think, a little bit of support for the hypothesis of ageing that I have favoured.

Undoubtedly there will be gerontologists with more ambition and more optimism than I have. Dr Defares, a Dutch gerontologist, is developing an approach to maintain a proper balance of hormones in the body for people of 50 and over, with a special concentration on the problems of post-menopausal women. There are suggestions that immune stimulation may be possible. In one talk I gave on ageing, to medical students, one of my audience made the logical, if at the moment impracticable, suggestion that, at about the age of 6, *half* the thymus should be removed and stored in liquid nitrogen until the child had passed through middle age. Then, when he was 60 or 65, transplant back his own thymus! Others might suggest the same procedure with bone marrow, or both bone marrow and thymus. I have no doubt, too, that if anti-oxidants are found to raise the Hayflick limit, they will be tested for possible effects in prolonging human life.

I am far from optimistic about the effectiveness of any of these suggested procedures and I have considerable worries about the ethics even of their experimental use. However, they will be tried. This makes a suggestion of Dr Alex Comfort's of special importance—that we should develop and apply objective tests for 'physiological' age. Everyone knows that some 65-year-olds are frail old men with physical and other signs of senility, whereas others are 'extraordinarily young for their age'. There are simple clinical and biochemical tests which can measure the physiological concomitants that allow us to judge a person's age. Proper application and analysis of such tests would first give us a firm background of what is normal in the community and then make it possible to prove the worthlessness of most recipes for longevity and, hopefully, to find some regime which does in fact slow down the process of senescence.

9

GENETIC ASPECTS OF
MENTAL DISEASE

It is self-evident that the genes we are born with provide, along with the rest of our functioning selves, the basis of our intelligence, temperament, and personality. They probably play a greater part than anything else which can be named in determining human behaviour, in all its range from the socially acceptable to the completely unacceptable, from consummate skill to utter clumsiness, and from intellectual genius to imbecility. Yet we have only to look at the matter slightly differently to say that a human being's inheritance, his genes, supply no more than the neural machinery on which the environment in its family, social, educational, and cultural aspects, will in more or less effective, more or less distorted, fashions build up the individual's pattern of behaviour and temperament. To come just a little closer to what matters most in a modern community, I like Washburn's formulation on the inheritance of instinct and behaviour; what we inherit is the capacity to learn a skill or an attitude, easily or with difficulty.

As every good teacher knows—or, for that matter, any experienced sergeant-major in the Army, any successful evangelist from John Wesley onwards, or any dedicated Communist—children and adults without any special desire or inherent ability to learn, can with skill and pressure be persuaded into learning almost anything and accepting without much difficulty, new cultural patterns. The educationalist and the psychologist make their point that within limits, and they are very wide limits, they can, given the means and the opportunity, bring most of the handicapped and the socially unacceptable to a condition of social usefulness and at least some degree of contentment to the individual.

There are limits, of course. At the lower end of the inherited ability to learn, whose expression is the level of measured IQ, there are the low-grade morons who can be taught to do simple repetitive work and conform amiably to any self-consistent social regime, but there are also groups lower still that are beyond the possibility of training. Mental deficiency is not mental disease but it is equally a deviation from the socially useful and acceptable.

To almost everyone, mental disease is something difficult to understand and embarrassing to confront. This holds at least as much for a laboratory scientist like myself, as for any one else. An attempt by one who is in no sense a psychiatrist, to say something useful about mental disease in the context of my general theme is perhaps unjustified. Except for a consideration of genetic and biochemical aspects of porphyria and schizophrenia, it can only provide a few impressions of the general problem presented by mental disease. Yet, mental disease and the emotional and neurotic concomitants of physical disease are so much a part of the human situation that confronts medical science that the topic can hardly be omitted.

One could start with the axiom that the definition of mental disease must be a social one. An individual needs the services of a psychiatrist if he suffers from a disabling intensity or duration of mood or, if through some loss of mental contact with reality, he cannot maintain an acceptable relationship to his community or accept responsibility for his own well-being.

It is clear that there is an enormous variety of manifestations of mental illness and that there is still no adequate way of classifying them into definiable diseases. Even an outsider can sense that nowhere can a line be drawn that will separate the normal from the mentally abnormal or decide unequivocally who is certifiable and who should remain in the community.

Perhaps the outstanding impression is the intimidating complexity of the human brain. The detail of thought and behaviour must in the last analysis depend on the circuitry of the brain and, if this is at fault, in mental disease there is no conceivable approach to repairing or replacing it. It may be that chemical aspects of the brain are equally complex but at least there is the possibility that they are more accessible. Consciously or unconsciously this may be part of the justification for the ruling hypothesis that biochemical processes are responsible for mood and its deviations. Especially with experience of the use of mood-controlling drugs, there seems to be more reason here for hope.

One gathers from limited reading in psychopathology that there are two constellations of major psychoses. The first, with frank schizophrenia as the type form, becomes evident usually between puberty and middle age with what is described as disintegration of the emotional stability of the patient—something which may take an unlimited range of individual forms. Occasionally the disease fails to progress with partial or rarely complete recovery but it usually goes on with progressive loss of contact with reality to complete dementia.

In the second group, phases of severe depression provide the major feature. In some individuals, with remission of the depression there is a swing of mood to elation, aggression, and instability that may reach manic level. This is the classical manic-depressive psychosis. The largest single group of certifiable patients are those suffering from the wide variety of senile and pre-senile dementias. Then there are all the personality patterns and the psychoneuroses that roughly represent the ways that vulnerable personalities break down under stress. It is a mere truism to say that every socially significant behavioural disorder has both genetic and environmental components while it is felt equally self-evident by most modern psychiatrists that all affective disorders—involving mood and emotion—are associated with biochemical changes in the brain.

THE CAUSATION OF MENTAL DISEASE

The social and emotional factors which are associated with, and perhaps responsible for mental disease and the psychosomatic disorders, are doubtless important but only in exceptional circumstances do the worries and conflicts which are claimed to be responsible, exceed those which most other individuals endure without breakdown. There seems to be no way in which a disease-producing episode can be recognized at anything more significant than an anecdotal level.

Within the current limitations of the scientific method there seem to be only three potentially rewarding approaches to understanding the cause—better the antecedents and triggering factors—of clinically significant disorders of behaviour and mood.

The first is to seek external causes of brain damage that could induce mental disease, trauma, infection, or a secondary result of disease elsewhere in the body. The second becomes evident when genetic investigations suggest that change in a *single gene* plays a dominant or exclusive role. The third approach is by the detection of some biochemical abnormality characteristic of the condition.

There are a number of ways in which definable causes from outside can precipitate mental symptoms. Traumatic brain damage as in the 'punch-drunk' boxer or the GPI (general paralysis of the insane) of chronic brain syphilis are classical examples. A brain tumour can produce mental symptoms, sometimes a tumour in the lung or elsewhere in the body can do the same. The very essence of drug addiction is its effect on the victim's behaviour. Prolonged use of amphetamine can bring some people into a schizophrenia-like condition; mescaline and LSD have their own characteristic effects on mood and behaviour, sometimes with hallucinations and dissociation from reality that resemble a schizophrenic condition. One of the drugs commonly used for high blood pressure, reserpine, can induce in some persons a profound depression. The potent effect of drugs reinforces the feeling amongst psychiatric investigators that the real basis of the psychoses is likely to be chemical rather than what could be called disorder in the circuitry of the brain.

In a slightly different sense, drugs may produce virtual insanity in persons genetically predisposed to respond to them.

PORPHYRIA

Porphyria is a name which covers a number of genetic diseases which result from chemical errors in handling the precursors of the blood pigments and characteristically produces a 'port wine'-coloured urine when fully manifest. Any of the forms can at times produce severe mental symptoms as part of the disease. At present the popular diagnosis of George III's recurrent bouts of insanity is that he suffered from inherited porphyria. In South Africa there are some thousands of persons carrying a gene for porphyria which has been shown quite convincingly to have come to the Cape of Good Hope in a single individual toward the end of the seventeenth century. The story of porphyria in South Africa has been pieced together into a fascinating book by Dr Geoffrey Dean and although its bearing on mental disease is rather marginal it has so many aspects relevant to the theme of this book that it is worth retelling at some length.

In his practice in Port Elizabeth, Dean became deeply interested in the genetic and other aspects of porphyria after treating a patient with a severe acute attack initiated, like most such episodes, by the use of barbiturate sleeping pills. He was aware that it was an inherited condition and was therefore particularly interested when his patient told him that it was well known that amongst the Afrikaans families related to her own, there was an inherited tendency to suffer from sensitive hands. The backs of the hands where they were exposed to sunlight tended to become inflamed and pigmented, a condition characteristic enough to be known by the name of the family as 'van Rooyen hands'. This was in fact the commonest symptom of South Africa porphyria giving it its name of porphyria variegata.

Any genetic condition recognizable by laymen as a family characteristic descending from father to son, must necessarily be a dominant one, its result being expressed to some degree in all who carry the abnormal gene. Almost invariably the affected individual will marry a spouse normal for the gene and the expectation will be that 50 per cent of children from such marriages will show the trait; $Aa \times aa$ gives Aa and aa in equal proportions.

Dean was first interested only in the van Rooyen clan but soon found himself involved in the mammoth task of tracing back the porphyria gene to its first appearance in South Africa. The early Boers were interested in their forbears and from parish registers, family traditions, and legal documents 1,120 persons diagnosed as porphyrics were traced back to one common ancestor. He was Gerrit Jansz who arrived at the Cape in 1685. Three years later he married one of eight girls sent out from a Dutch orphanage to provide wives for the pioneer settlers. They had a large family (8); one son-in-law was a van Rooyen of the 'hands' and the progenitor of a large clan. Three other of their children were carriers of the gene which must have come either from Gerrit or his wife, Ariantje.

Dean calculates from limited surveys of individuals for signs of porphyria and the distribution of the relevant surnames that there are probably 8,000 white South Africans plus a few 'coloureds' now carrying the gene. The implication that a single gene could multiply to this extent in less than 300 years is something unique in human population genetics but it is supported by genealogical data on the Dutch in South Africa. The surnames of the forty free burghers who settled in the Cape around 1685 are now held by approximately one million of the Afrikaaner people. This gives a general rate of increase of the same order as that of the couple who introduced the gene. It is clear that the fertility of the Dutch pioneers was extraordinarily high, mainly in the sense of a survival of children to adulthood that was unique for that period of history. One can assume with certainty that their survival was basically due to the almost complete absence of infectious disease. The land was almost empty of indigenous inhabitants. Most of the Hottentots had died of the smallpox that came with the Dutch. The farming life was healthy and for twelve to sixteen children to survive to adulthood was common. More land was always available and Dean is probably correct in saying that the situation was unique in the population expansion that it allowed. In Europe there was a six-fold increase in 300 years; in South Africa, 12,500-fold.

Obviously the dominant gene for porphyria was no serious handicap to those who carried it and even now it would do 'them little harm if it had not been for modern medicine' to quote Dean's words. Acute porphyria is a condition with a high mortality whose symptoms are severe abdominal pain, a highly emotional state which can pass into frank hysteria or be associated with hallucinations and delusions of persecution, and progressive paralysis. It is more severe in women than in men, and is *always* associated with the taking of drugs, usually barbiturates, sometimes sulphonamides. The essence of the situation is that the genetic defect as such has no influence on behaviour but it provides a background that allows an otherwise harmless drug to produce acute mental and physical disease. There are a number of other genetic conditions that can make other drugs a lethal hazard to the individual but they have no relevance to mental disease. The importance of porphyria is the possibility that it may serve as a model for the still indefinite genetic basis of schizophrenia.

SCHIZOPHRENIA

No competent psychiatrist seems to have any doubt that there is at least a strong genetic predisposition to schizophrenia or that it is associated with some biochemical abnormality. In neither the genetic or the biochemical field is it possible to make any definitive statement of the position and there are still authorities who look for psychosocial difficulties as being the responsible trigger.

The simplest statement of the genetic position is to say that schizophrenia is dependent on the presence of a dominant gene with about 25 per cent 'penetrance' (100 per cent penetrance means that a gene always shows its presence: 0 per cent penetrance means that it never does). A fully dominant gene would mean that a schizophrenic married to a normal spouse should have 50 per cent of children with the disease. Actual figures show that children from families with one schizophrenic parent will develop schizophrenia at a much lower frequency ranging from 10 to 18 per cent in different investigations. This gives a measure of the so-called penetrance of the gene. On the other hand it must also be noted that 60 per cent of schizophrenic patients give no family history whatever of this illness. There seems to be no doubt that in some families the incidence of the disease points to a dominant gene of relatively high penetrance. For the rest, all that can be said is that genetic constitution plays a part which cannot yet be properly evaluated.

Much the same conclusion has come from the application of the classical twin study method. As in all such investigations the objective was to obtain as many subjects as possible with the condition, who had a twin. In general, twins occur about once every sixty or seventy births so that in a common condition like schizophrenia, reasonably large numbers of such index twins can be found. In each case the 'other' twin is examined, first to determine whether the twin pair is 'identical' (monozygous, formed from a single fertilized egg) or 'non-identical' (dizygous, formed from two separate fertilized eggs), and second, for the abnormal quality, in this case, schizophrenia. In the first major investigation made by Kallmann in 1938, his results showed that when monozygotic identical twins were examined, the other twin was also schizophrenic in 86 per cent of cases, i.e., there was 86 per cent concordance. With non-identical dizygotic twins and ordinary siblings of the index twin, the concordance was only around 15 per cent. In subsequent studies where the diagnosis of schizophrenia has been made more critically the degree of concordance has been much lower, 30–42 per cent in identical twins, 9 per cent in non-identical. The most recent study I have seen, published in 1970, analysed a set of identical twins one of whom, the 'index twin', was diagnosed as definite schizophrenia. In this group the second twins showed schizophrenia, i.e., concordance, in 44 per cent. Another

TWINS

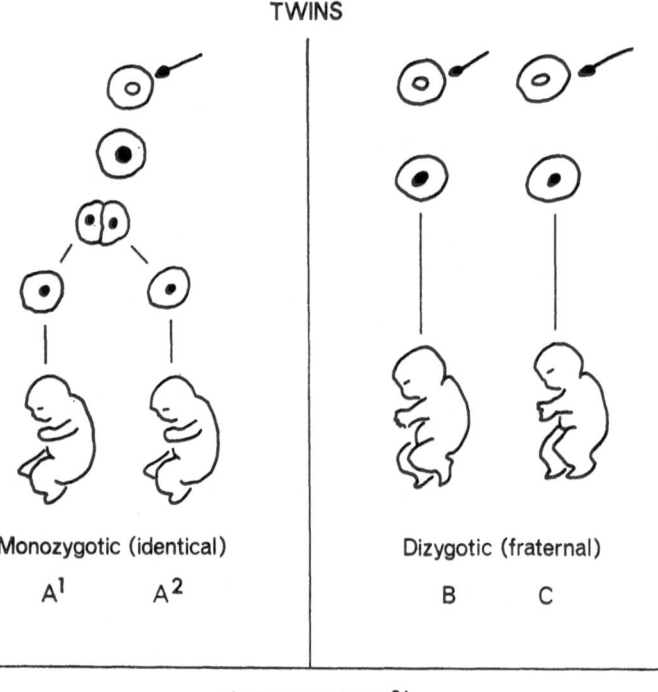

CONCORDANCE %

Genetic origin	100	20 ±
Environmental	20 ±	20 ±
Mixed	50	20

FIG. 42. To illustrate the use of identical and fraternal twins in differentiating between genetic and environmental effects. From a large group of persons with disease X, those who were born as twins are selected as 'index cases'. Their twins are located and it is decided from physical and blood group examinations whether they are identical one-egg twins or non-identical. The proportion of second twins with disease X gives the degree of concordance. When the concordance in identical twins is significantly higher than with dissimilar twins, a genetic component is playing a part in causing the disease.

43 per cent were diagnosed as showing schizoid personality and the remaining 13 per cent were normal.

No one has satisfactorily interpreted these results. Clearly, inheritance does no more than provide a strong predisposition toward schizophrenic breakdown. The trigger that sets the process in motion is as obscure as the nature of the process itself. It is reasonably certain that in some families at least, a single dominant gene is necessary but it is equally clear that the primary effect of the gene does not produce schizophrenia. From the identical twin results, the secondary trigger factors cannot be genetic. There have been suggestions that somatic mutation and auto-immune processes may act as a trigger and there is the possibility that something absorbed from the intestine could act in a way remotely like the action of barbiturate in a person with latent porphyria. By far the most popular suggestion is that the additional factor needed is social and psychological stress but, again, there is no light thrown on either the trigger or the basis of the developed disease.

Probably more interest has been directed to the possible bio-chemical basis of schizophrenia than to either of the other approaches.

Circumstantial evidence points rather strongly in that direction but one gathers that there is still unresolved controversy over the view that the one-time famous 'pink spot' seen on chromatographs from the urine of schizophrenics is characteristic of the disease. There is good evidence that disturbance in the metabolism of 'mono-amines' such as serotonin and noradrenalin (epinephrine) is present in the schizophrenic. These are substances with a physiological role in the conduction of nerve impulses from one cell to another in the brain. The drug mescaline, used for centuries by Nevadan and Mexican Indians to produce hallucinations and mood change, is chemically quite closely related to the physiological mono-amines and the pink spot was ascribed to a derivative of noradrenaline, much closer still to mescaline. Even if the pink spot is found much more frequently in schizophrenics than in other individuals it does not, of course, follow that the substance responsible for the spot on the test paper is what causes the symptoms of the disorder. It could just as readily be a secondary result of some quite distinct metabolic anomaly.

My only conclusion is that no one has produced a satisfactory understanding of schizophrenia. Genetic factors obviously play a part and in the developed disease there are definite metabolic abnormalities associated with and probably, in part, responsible for abnormalities of neural conduction in the brain. Stochastic analysis of the age incidence of first admission to treatment for schizophrenia is used by Burch to support the idea that some autoimmune process provides the essential trigger. As in so many other contexts, one wonders whether the most important difficulty, to the understanding of schizophrenia, is not the sheer complexity of the situation. The uniqueness of every human personality, the genetic and developmentally derived diversity of brain circuitry, and the established complexity of the way amines, etc., become concerned physiologically in nerve conduction from cell to cell, each resists from its nature the scientific approach. I should predict with some confidence that, though the future will undoubtedly see new and relevant discoveries, they will not significantly diminish the incidence of schizophrenia.

Porphyria and schizophrenia are the only diseases that it would be justifiable to discuss in the context of this book. Even less is known about the other main conditions which bring people into the mental hospitals, and treatment for them all remains basically empirical.

THE SOCIAL PROBLEM

It is conventional to emphasize the size of the mental illness problem and the need for research in this field. In most advanced countries something of the order of half the total hospital beds are occupied by mental patients. In England and Wales a fairly recent estimate of the numbers of persons requiring care and treatment as a result of mental deficiency or disease approached one million. It was made up of persons with certifiable mental disease, 3 per 1,000, about 6 per 1,000 mentally deficient individuals and a proportion that may amount to 1 per cent of the population with psychoneurotic illness or disability. It is an accepted community objective that those suffering from, or handicapped by, mental disability should be brought back to a state of social usefulness and personal happiness in so far as that is possible in the current state of knowledge. It is a task of overwhelming size which could never be achieved even in principle unless care of the afflicted became the full-time business of a quite disporportionate number of the most intelligent people in the community. Every psychiatrist can cite examples of intensely rewarding responses to intelligent care but one gathers that in the great majority the factors which determine spontaneous recovery or progression to dementia are still unknown and treatment correspondingly empirical.

The development of drugs which can modify the basic symptoms of mental disease, anxiety, tension, depression, and hyperexcitability, has been extremely valuable in reducing the necessity for institutional care and for the use of drastic last resort types of treatment such as surgical leucotomy or electro-convulsive therapy. No one can doubt that the more humane, less restrictive regime of a good modern hospital is highly desirable, or that when an intelligent enthusiast has scope for application of his own ideas—whether based on psycho-analysis, group therapy, or learning theory or almost anything else—to the rehabilitation of his patients, they will do better than average. The various institutions that come under a mental health authority need more staff and higher-quality personnel at all levels. But the reality must be faced that to the vast majority of ordinary people, care of the mentally abnormal is unattractive and to obtain and hold sufficient suitable staff to give individual care to patients who could benefit from it may never be practicable. The over-all results will always be capable of improvement but there will always be a very large, hard core of socially unassimilable individuals.

At the level of research, one can only be pessimistic even about long-term prospects. Everyone has a skeleton in his cupboard, which can be translated as 'a certain burden of genes which in some reshuffle will result in the birth of a descendant predestined for mental illness'. Having regard both to recessive genes and dominant genes of low penetrance there is no approach visible to the prevention of mental disease by eugenic or other measures. Schizophrenia is certain to remain a major target for research and here one can feel a faint optimism that biochemical or immunological approaches ought eventually to allow us to understand the trigger which at a certain time in life sets the disease process in action. If the basic condition in schizophrenia is a definable biochemical abnormality there might conceivably be opportunities to seek a chemotherapeutic approach. Nothing hopeful seems to be available at present and there can be no certainty that even a greatly increased understanding of schizophrenia would allow us to control or cure it.

10

THE POPULATION PROBLEM

In the last year or two we have become used to seeing colour photographs of the Earth in space. With its colours of seas and continents and its broken swirls of cloud cover, it presents an extraordinary contrast to what can be seen on the moon or Mars. We have known it all along but now it is laid out for all to see. The Earth is a sphere of finite size and unique as an abode for man. We have nowhere else to go.

Man is the dominant organism on the earth and unless he or his descendant species are completely exterminated there is no possibility that any other organism can evolve to contest that dominance. It is likely, then, that we and our descendant species will control the same planet and nothing more for the 3, 4, or 5 thousand million years that, barring some cosmic catastrophe, are available while the sun continues to supply energy at the rate which keeps the Earth habitable. I regard it as self-evident that 'eventually' we must develop a stable human ecosystem for the Earth. Last year I wrote a book[1] to underline that necessity and to repeat what many others are thinking but few are saying, that every measure of what we are doing points inexorably toward chaos and catastrophe within a century—unless we can accept, understand, and work effectively toward the self-evident necessity.

Basically I agree with the pessimists that current civilization will destroy itself and that a second scientific civilization rebuilt in centuries or millennia from pockets of survivors will probably again end in utter catastrophe. Yet, at the emotional level, neither I nor any other intelligent human being can accept so hopeless a forecast. I believe that the only thing that really matters in the next twenty years—we may not even have as long as that—is to produce a climate of world opinion and blueprints for progressive action that will bring us to the first crude and unstable form of a global human ecosystem.

1. *Dominant Mammal*, Heinemann, Melbourne.

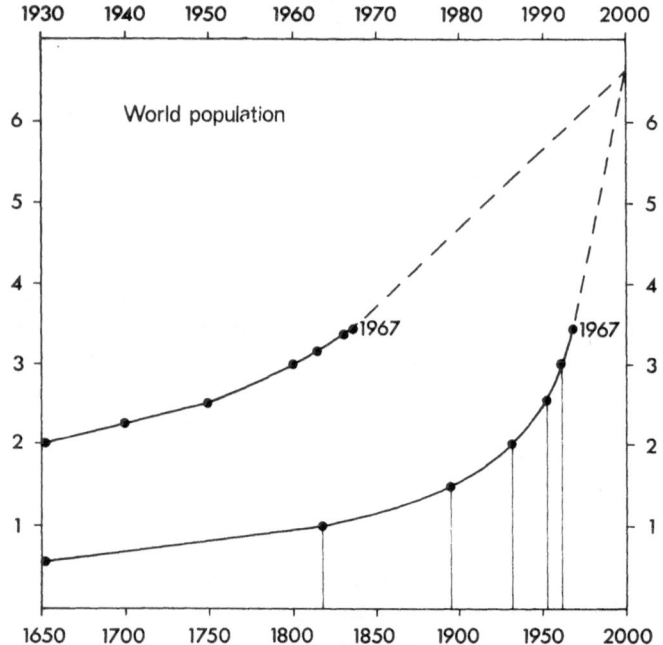

FIG. 43. World population and its extrapolation to A.D. 2000. Two time-scales are shown, the upper in decades since 1930, and the lower in half-centuries since 1650. The vertical scale is in thousand millions and vertical lines show when each successive addition of 500 million was reached. (*Dominant Mammal.*)

There are countless intractable problems at the level of social, economic, and political requirements but the biological aspects are basic and they are the only ones I can be concerned with in a book about genes. The first requirement for a stable human ecosystem is the maintenance of a population level that the Earth can support from its indefinitely renewable resources. Everyone is well aware that at the present time, world population is doubling every thirty years. At this rate there will be 7,000 million in 2000; 14 billion in 2030; 60 billion in 2100; and about 7×10^{18} (7,000 million billions) in the year 3000, which is only as far ahead of us as Alfred the Great is behind us. The calculation is, of course, quite absurd but so far no one has shown how to bring the world rate of increase quickly down to the zero, ± 0.5 per cent per annum, that is needed.

Even the optimists can see no real possibility of avoiding growth to the 20 billion level before stabilization can be reached. In 1971 we are approaching the 4 billion mark and it seems an over-crowded and unhappy, polluted and plundered world. With five times the number it will be much more than five times worse. When we calculate that fossil fuels will be exhausted by 3000 AD and that the inevitable replacement by nuclear energy will, more slowly than an atomic war but just as surely in the long run, poison the whole Earth with radiation, we come on another biological imperative. That the stable human population must in the end make do with the energy provided by the sun and used very close to the time it is received. The sun is the only large-scale source of energy whose use does not exhaust the supply or pollute the environment. Given the direction and the necessity, solar energy can be exploited in water and wind power, timber as fuel and by conversion of solar radiation to heat and electricity by some rela-tively direct method. Once methods of placing large collectors of solar energy in geostationary orbit and beaming energy to the Earth's surface are developed, a considerable increase in popula-tion could be envisaged. As things are, the reasonable level would probably be between 1 and 2 billion people, less than half our present numbers, but about the same number as in 1920.

There is only one socially important objective for medical research or scholarly work in sociology, economics, or politics in 1971. This is to find the techniques and make it economically, politically, and psychologically possible to apply them, which will allow the world's population to be stabilized within a hundred years at 2 billion or whatever other equilibrium level is found to be appropriate. Nothing else has anything like this importance. Even the more widely realized necessity to remove the possibility of full-scale nuclear war must take second place. Any general appreciation of the ecological situation of man would make nuclear war henceforth unthinkable. Failure to act on population will bring mounting disorders and all the psychoses of power whose only logical outcome is the suicidal use of the world's arsenal of doomsday weapons.

AN OUTLINE OF HUMAN EVOLUTION

In this chapter I want to write about those aspects of human population that seem relevant, even if it is only rather distantly relevant, to the theme of this book. That theme is basically the medical problems that remain when we brush aside the successful elimination in the affluent world of disease due to the impact of the environment, and the reasons why disease based on genetic anomaly at either germinal or somatic level is so much more difficult to prevent or treat.

What will need to be discussed are the changing nature of the limitations on population that were effective in human prehistory and history, the evolution of the main human races, the relationship of infectious disease to the development of urban life, and finally the impact of the industrial and scientific revolutions.

There seems to be general agreement that the evolution of man took place from primates that were widely spread over Africa and Asia and that the first definite hominoid fossils are of the Australopithecines of South and East Africa about 2 million years ago. These had brains no larger than a gorilla's but walked upright on two feet and probably used simple weapons and tools of wood and bone. In all probability the change from small groups similar to those of gorilla and chimpanzee to the only slightly larger groups of food-gatherers and hunters was gradual over the 2 million years which included the whole of the Pleistocene glacial period. It is assumed that at any time during those long ages the human population was widely distributed in small bands over the unglaciated parts of the Old World, that there was considerable variability in physical type but sufficient interbreeding between groups to maintain an open gene pool. With the possible exception of the appearance and disappearance of Neanderthal man, no separate species of man ever emerged. As judged by the rarity of human fossils the numbers of early man probably remained roughly constant over the long term but would inevitably be subject to gross local fluctuations. Mortality must have been consistently high, probably for the most part by physical mishap. This would include attack by beasts of prey and injuries while hunting, or in battle with other groups; death by flood, fire, and famine must also have been frequent. Infectious disease specific to the human species probably was almost nonexistent when aggregations were limited to small wandering bands. When, however, a group moved after long residence in high temperate country to low-level swamps and jungles with much mammalian and bird life and numerous biting insects, they would almost certainly find themselves susceptible to one or other of the protozoal or virus parasites being spread through the animals of the area. If a human population was to develop that could exploit such areas, it needed to develop a capacity for its young to become harmlessly immunized against the prevalent pathogens.

Any population of food-gatherers will be subject to the sort of situation appropriate for the phenomenon of genetic drift which appears to have been an important feature of human evolution. This occurs when a very small unit, in the limit one man and one woman, becomes isolated from all other populations for sufficient time to allow its descendants to multiply to a substantial group.

In any large population that is able to mate more or less at random the various genetic characters by which people differ from one another, their blood groups, for example, become distributed in a pattern which remains approximately constant for the group. With an 'Adam and Eve' situation, however, the founding couple will carry only a small sample of all the genes that were available in their original population. Until mutation becomes significant, all their descendants, however, will be limited to various recombinations of their genes and no others. The eventual result will be a new population with some relatively uniform characteristic not shown by any other group. Anomalies of blood group distribution provide the most easily demonstrated examples. North Greenland Eskimos, for instance, possess only group O. Drift could, however, be equally relevant in relation to less precise aspects. Gajdusek has described an isolated Pacific atoll where the population is grossly below the average standard of intelligence of their race and at the other end of the scale it is hard to imagine how otherwise than through genetic drift the concentration of genius in Athens of the fourth century BC could have arisen.

The evolution and distribution of human qualities must have been quite exceptionally complicated for a mammalian species. In particular the existence of geologically rapid changes of climate— four glacial epochs and three interglacial warm periods in 1·5 million years—plus the capacity of men to modify their own 'climate' by the invention of clothing and shelter interacted to allow the occupation of a wide range of territory with increasing possibility of small or large groups becoming isolated from others for very long periods. The major racial groups, negroid, caucasoid, mongoloid, and australoid, probably became differentiated by isolation. In the opposite direction the specifically human cultural pattern of war probably did much to assure a continuing flow of genes between races. The standard pattern, presumably from the earliest phases of human culture, was to kill as many adult males of the 'enemy' as possible but to mate with their women. Even if the progeny were initially underprivileged they were 'within the gene pool' and all the important genes of the conquered were now potentially available for new recombinations. This is probably what is mainly responsible for the lack of any sharp demarcations as one moves from one centre to another of the three racial types of the Old World.

THE ROLE OF INFECTIOUS DISEASE

Infectious disease amongst wild animals and birds is only very rarely a major cause of mortality. There is an infinite range of parasites from viruses to worms which live at their expense but do not usually produce frank disease. Only the infections of wild animals which produce human disease have been investigated in any depth. The plague bacillus has its ancestral home with the burrowing tarbagans of the Siberian steppes and has managed to find new hosts in South Africa (gerbilles) and in California (ground squirrels). In all, the infection remains virtually invisible for most of the time but for reasons unknown, widespread fatal outbreaks in the host species occur from time to time. In Australia, psittacosis is widespread in wild parrots and cockatoos but only once (in 1937) has there been evidence of extensive fatal psittacosis amongst wild birds. The mosquito-borne viruses of the tropics which produce a variety of human fevers, with yellow fever the most serious, are all derived from animal reservoirs and with occasional exceptions, such as yellow fever in some South American monkeys, the animal carriers are not seriously affected.

Small groups of wandering food-gatherers would never be in a position to generate infectious diseases specific to man. Just as plague can maintain itself only in gregarious species like rats and tarbagans, infectious disease became a significant factor in human evolution only with the beginnings of urban life and civilization. The first cities were in the subtropical regions of the Middle East and India and civilization moved soon into the tropics proper. Everything suggests that specifically human infections which were to become the main controller of human populations, evolved chiefly in the tropics.

In the wet tropics with a high mean temperature and abundant rain, all life moves at a faster tempo and when the rain-forest ecosystem was in equilibrium, the whole turnover was at a higher level than in temperate regions. Plants grew more rapidly, animals and birds of all types were more abundant, there were hosts of organisms to turn dead organic material swiftly into a form which would make its nitrogen and phosphorus again available for plant growth. The evolution of flying insects living by blood-sucking provided an ecological niche to be exploited by parasites of many types, of which malaria was to become the most humanly important. It is self-evident that the more closely packed the host population the more readily will a parasite move from infected to previously uninfected individuals. It is equally obvious that a parasite which kills every animal it infects will soon become extinct.

With the development of tropical agriculture, urban development, and concomitantly the evolution of an increasing variety of human infectious disease, a new ecological balance came into being in which human fertility was countered by infectious disease, particularly by its effect on infantile mortality. Over-all, a reasonably stable population with average annual deaths equal to births, could be expected in an area large enough to be representative and to allow for immigration into the cities from the country and other internal movements. There are chronic infections which lower fertility, such as malaria and gonorrhoea but even so, the birth-rate in an unsophisticated community will be close to the physiological maximum which is probably about 60 per 1,000 per annum. Taking a value of 40 for the birth-rate and a similar value for the death-rate, the standard expectation of life at birth would be around twenty-five years. Unless this is recognized clearly as merely a useful abstraction for demographers it is liable to mislead. People do not die on the average around the age of 25 in such a community. The great majority of deaths are in infancy and childhood and once an individual has, as it were, run the gauntlet of infectious disease and reached adult life, he is likely to survive to 50 or 60.

In all probability a similar situation held in most of the world's cities at least until the beginning of the eighteenth century. It was well known that the cities always had to be replenished by the excess of young people who survived in the less-crowded, healthier countryside. A specially pertinent example of the extent of human proliferative potential in the absence of infectious disease has already been quoted in relation to the spread of porphyria in South Africa. The pioneer Afrikaners had a population doubling time of about twenty years, giving an increase of 12,500-fold in just less than 300 years.

In the move from the food-gathering to the agricultural and urban economy there was a progressive slow increase in numbers but the excess of births over deaths was always very small by modern standards. The principal causes of death changed from accident and hardship to infection, but at all stages there was a reasonably stabilized human ecosystem. In all communities it was necessary for the birth-rate to be high enough to make good the mortality but not to do more. Cultural practices to reduce the birth-rates, such as taboos on intercourse during a prolonged period of lactation after each birth, might be needed to lower the birth-rate below the physiological maximum. In such cultures any breakdown of tradition would, other things being equal, bring back the birth-rate to the maximum. At the genetic level the evolutionary programming of human reproductive life, to run from 15 to 45 years of age with old age starting about 60, was probably established in the near 2 million years of food-gathering. All the modifications in the last 5,000–7,000 years must have been essentially cultural.

The accelerating increase of human populations since the beginning of the eighteenth century have depended mainly on two factors, an increase in the amount of food available and the development, incidentally or deliberately, of ways of diminishing infectious disease. The conscious development of science for human benefit can be reasonably dated from the mid seventeenth century when the Royal Society and the European academies were founded. All the factors leading to population increase were deeply influenced by the scientific and technical advances of the last 300 years. The improvement of agricultural methods in Europe and the selection of superior varieties of food plants became important in the seventeenth century. In the eighteenth century, the European colonization of the empty lands overseas began, aided by improvements in ships and the science of navigation, while in Europe the construction of canals greatly cheapened the transport of food to where it was needed. The industrial revolution began to bring more people into the cities and worsened the slums but with the increased output of goods that came as factories multiplied there was a steady rise in the standard of living of all classes. This in itself tended automatically to diminish the prevalence of at least some forms of infectious disease.

Any improvement in cleanliness and comfort has been regarded as desirable from the beginnings of history. Ruling classes have usually seen to it that they had baths and could wear freshly laundered clothing, that no sight or smell of excreta should persist in their dwellings, that water should be clear and free of taint, and that food should be fresh and appetizing. Without any knowledge of bacteriology at all, action which extended comforts of this sort down the social scale automatically improved the chances of survival. In England the first Public Health Act in 1848, setting up requirements and responsibilities for the provision of pure water supplies and proper disposal of sewage, was the beginning of regularized control that was soon given a rationale and a new effectiveness with the recognition of bacteria as agents of diseases. The effect of deliberate interference of the state in public health matters plus the rising standard of living can be seen in the steady increase in population in Europe during the second half of the nineteenth century. Medical science was moving ahead with more and more confidence. Hospitals became places where patients could hope to recover, instead of the pestilential centres for septic infections of every sort that they had been. It is doubtful whether a direct effect on demographic statistics could be claimed for civilian measures deliberately based on the medical sciences until the 1920s. Diphtheria immunization and the use of insulin for the treatment of diabetes brought the first of the large-scale effects of specifically based action against disease to supplement the general benefits to health of a rising standard of living. From then on there was a fantastic third of a century which, by allowing in principle complete control of infectious disease throughout the world, changed the whole pattern of history. It suddenly became clear that history had always been concerned with the changes in the numbers and distribution of human beings with time but had never realized that infectious disease and food supply were more important than wars and politics. The sulpha drugs, the anti-

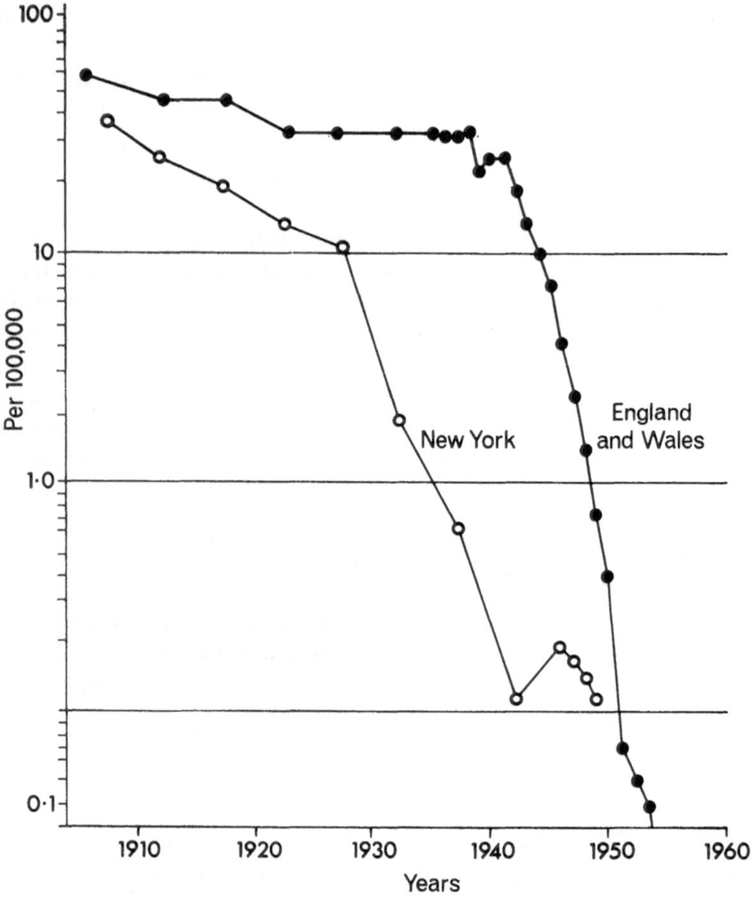

FIG. 44. The effect of immunization on deaths from diphtheria in Britain and in the United States. (*Natural History of Infectious Disease*, Cambridge University Press.)

biotics, DDT, and the other potent insecticides, anti-malarial drugs and those that could cure tuberculosis and leprosy, immunization against whooping cough, polio, tetanus and measles, yellow fever and typhus—these and the principles for their large-scale application have changed a steady population increase into an explosion.

The classical example of the effect specific action against an

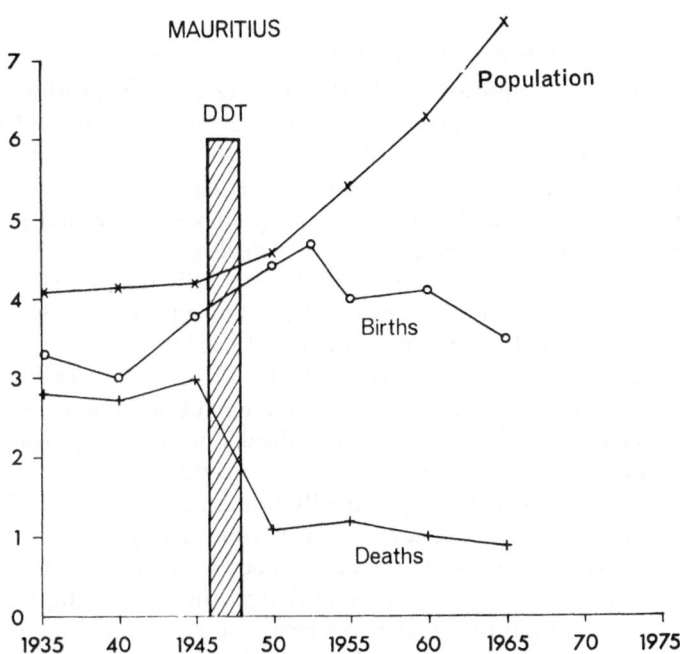

F IG. 45. The influence of malaria eradication on the demography of Mauritius. Malaria was eradicated around 1946–8. The bar marks the period when *Anopheles gambiense* and *A. funestus* were eliminated. Population in hundred thousands. Birth- and death-rates per 100 per annum. (*Dominant Mammal.*)

infectious disease can have on the vital statistics of a community is still the result of eliminating malarial mosquitoes and therefore malaria from Mauritius in 1946–8. During the war years, death-rates were around 30 per 1,000 per annum, birth-rates about 33, giving a slow increase in population somewhat below 0·5 per cent per annum. After 1948 the whole pattern changed. The birth-rate rose to 48 and infantile mortality fell to 80 from its former level of 150; general death-rate fell precipitately to 15. Subsequently the birth-rate has diminished a little but birth and death-rates have stayed widely apart and the island's population has soared from 300,000 to 800,000 in twenty years. Mauritius is still only 720 square miles in area.

THE POSSIBILITIES OF POPULATION CONTROL

The world is in approximately the same state as Mauritius with population expanding at close to 2 per cent per annum and vast areas of malarious country still unreclaimed. The elimination of infectious disease was as disastrously short-sighted as the creation of the atomic bomb. Both were equally inevitable results in the last analysis of the seventeenth-century decision to develop science for human benefit. It was always and necessarily human benefit in the short term as interpreted by the ruling group of one's own country in the light of their own cultural background.

The problem now is to reverse the trend, while it remains unthinkable not to continue the elimination of infectious disease wherever we can. When we think medically or demographically, it is accepted that sex and survival are the right of every man and woman, though it is perhaps equally human in other contexts to praise the virtues of celibacy and martyrdom and *pro patria mori*. The problem of consciously separating sex from reproduction has been solved for those with the knowledge, the purchasing power, and the motivation to use the contraceptive devices available. On the positive side is the universal recognition by women in affluent societies that a small family, or even no family, can allow a more enjoyable life than twenty or more years of closely spaced pregnancies. This, however, must be qualified by the common decision by women who use contraception intelligently that four children is the best size for a small family—and four children is two too many today. Family planning with its slogan of the children you want when you want them, is totally inadequate; it is population control or chaos.

On the negative side we have every religious or political group which believes it will add to its power or status if its numbers can be increased at a greater rate than for those outside the group. This includes the Roman Catholic Church, and many other less prestigious Christian sects, black activists in America—'Breed, baby, breed!'—and probably a host of power groups that we hear little or nothing about. The Communist powers have never firmly accepted the principle of population control but then Japan and India are the only sovereign powers that have. Australia has a blatantly expansionist population policy.

Clearly, motivation is the important aspect of population control, both at the individual and the general cultural level. Acceptance by governments and religious hierarchies will to some extent be determined by the breadth of the demand at lower levels but conversely they may effectively block the development of any demand. There is no justification for any attempt to discuss political and religious obstructions to population control at length in the present context. What seems specially relevant to my general approach is the relationship of medical care in the developing countries to the *control* of the population explosion as well as being the main cause of the problem.

MEDICAL NEEDS OF DEVELOPING COUNTRIES

There is a saying of Bernard Shaw's which can be relevant in many contexts that biological necessities must be made respectable; in other words, that cultural patterns are adapted to the needs for survival over the period in which the patterns were developed. From the standpoint of a peasant farmer in Asia or Africa, children are important as helpers in the field, as a means of ensuring that the land he occupies will remain 'in the family', and probably most of all because adult children will contribute to his support in old age. The overriding requirement is a son who will survive to maturity. This may well develop into the main obstacle to the acceptance of population control policies. With the knowledge that in the past anything from 20 to 50 per cent of children born failed to reach maturity, the feeling is natural that a family of four or five with at least two boys is necessary to provide security for the parents' old age. Action by a majority along these lines would, of course, only expand the dimensions of the population explosion. The only moves which could counter this attitude must be such as to provide credible security within the limitations necessitated by control of population. The provision of pensions by the welfare state is not likely to reach the villages for many years. In the meantime the need is to provide an environment which will increase the expectation of life at birth by at least halving infant mortality and providing preventive and curative medicine for the children to near Western standards.

At times I have felt that the only hope of fulfilling the need that village people should believe with reason that if they have only two children both will survive to maturity, was by supporting a massive increase in the number of medical schools so that in the minimum time something approaching 1 medical graduate per 1,000 of population will be available. In the long run this may become necessary, but the high status of the doctor in Western countries will always make it difficult for a graduate in a developing country to accept the lower status and salary that would go with a village practitioner's position. One gathers from the published figures that very large numbers of Indian and Pakistani medical graduates emigrate at the first opportunity to the United States or Britain. Indian village practice is the last thing they would be interested in.

Everything that I have heard of the practice of medicine in non-Communist developing countries indicates that it is almost impossible to attract a medical practitioner to undertake village work when there are available better-paid positions in the more attractive city environments. This is said not to hold in Communist countries but even in Russia it is admitted that every ambitious physician or surgeon wants to work in Moscow. The solution may well be to use local personnel at a much lower level of education than a medical degree acceptable in England or the United States.

It may well become urgent that the developing countries should swing from their current policy that the medical practitioner needs to have upper-class status and salary and must be educated to the same standards as are traditional in the West. The USSR may provide a better model where there is an accepted grade of *feldscher* capable of routine and first-aid activities as well as a very large number of medical practitioners most of whom are women with salaries in the upper bracket of skilled artisans. Around 1965 there were 443,000 medical practitioners and 364,100 medical assistants in the USSR. There is also, of course, a small upper stratum of hospital administrators, specialist physicians and surgeons, professors and heads of the research institutes of the Academy of Medical Sciences.

One gathers from the reports of recent discussions that the ideal system is to produce an infrastructure of large numbers of medical assistants, nurses, midwives, and birth control technicians, salaried and under discipline, and trained only to do efficiently and by a standardized technique the routine requirements of each community. These requirements are:

1. Education in and supervision of the appropriate method of birth control;

2. Antenatal and obstetric care by midwives;

3. Immunizations of children;

4. Standard treatment for infections;

5. Recognition of malnutrition and simple advice to remedy it;

6. Treatment of common non-lethal injuries according to standard rules.

Adequate supervision by senior personnel with higher-level training is essential and the whole structure demands at the top a system of medical training colleges which can bring the various curricula and teaching methods constantly into an effective relationship with the changing requirements in the field.

It would be conventional and humanitarian to add that the field personnel should all be able to recognize when a person required more advanced treatment than they were competent to provide and that such patients should be transferred immediately by ambulance or helicopter to an adequately staffed and equipped base hospital. This, however, will always be stage 2 or stage 3.

For a long time in every developing country there will be circumstances where death which could be averted if conditions of medical care were ideal, is inevitable.

It will have been noticed that everything which has been suggested is concerned only with the 'impact of the environment', the prevention and treatment of infectious disease and malnutrition, and the treatment of injury. If this is done with reasonably full effectiveness the rest can be left with confidence to the traditional practitioners of medicine and magic, and the general customs and common sense of the community. With every advance in education and living standard, things will move toward the Western standard of medical care or, one might hope, to something even better able to maintain health and less concerned with the status of the practitioner. For the immediate future, however, I believe that there is no real need for a developing country to concern itself beyond its own traditional ways with psychoses and psychoneuroses nor with the degenerations or diseases of old age including cancer, and even less with rare inherited disabilities becoming evident in infancy.

In other words I am excluding from the requirements of medicine in the expanding less affluent countries, everything with which this book is primarily concerned. And I believe that despite the length of what, as I have just implied, is a chapter of irrelevancies, the point does add something to the atmosphere of understanding that I should like to create.

We come back to the thesis that the overriding requirements in the 1970s are the spread of effective population control throughout the world, in affluent countries as well as in the poverty-stricken regions of the tropics, and the necessary corollary that people in the developing areas should have a sense that the two children the state will limit them to, will survive to make secure their parents' old age.

Quite obviously it is impossible to discuss the interrelated problems in every developing country, of the medical care of children and the provision of advice on and facilities for contraception, in more than very general terms without a local and contemporary knowledge of the position. It is only too clear that the move to stabilized population control will be of extreme difficulty and far slower than the situation demands. General education, education in the need for population control, propaganda on the personal advantage of having a small family, monetary incentives for surgical sterilization, they are all needed. Possibly more important still is a rising standard of living with some time for leisure to think. One ends with gloomy certainty that the little I have seen of developing countries and most of what I have read indicates that no democratic political machine will ever undertake an effective policy of population control. The only qualification to that statement involves the unlikely contingency of world recognition that the condition is so desperate that population control at existing levels must be made a national objective in every country including the great powers themselves, and that its achievement must be aided by every type of technical help, financial and other types of aid and even, if necessary, sanctions against non-co-operation.

11

AIMS AND LIMITATIONS OF THERAPY

I started to write this book with the objective of looking critically at what I regard as extravagant claims about the possibility of curing disease or changing human quality by 'genetic engineering'. This committed me to an attempt to look at the present situation and future prospects of the enlarging area of medical care which is concerned with things not associated with the impact of the environment on the body. With infection, malnutrition, and trauma put on one side there still remain first, the disorders with a large component of social impact, the psychoneuroses and the psychosomatic illnesses. Then come the intrinsic causes of disability and disease, genetic abnormality at the germ-cell level, somatic mutation in all its forms and the only partially unravelled complex of ageing and degenerative disease. What seems to have emerged from that discussion is that nowhere have useful means of rectifying these abnormalities or degenerations within the limits of the normal, been found. There are remedies galore, some of which, like surgery for malignant disease, may be sometimes curative in the full sense, others which by prolonging life or providing symptomatic relief, are fully accepted as necessary and valuable.

To complete the current picture, one must add the large amount of iatrogenic illness resulting from treatment applied in good faith and sometimes in the first instance, actually life-saving. It is disturbing to find in a hospital ward gross hormonal imbalance with 'moonface' and sometimes mental changes (caused by cortisone, etc.), acute allergic symptoms sometimes lethal (caused by penicillin, serums), paralysis of the bone marrow (caused by chloramphenicol and, less commonly, many other drugs), lupoid disease (caused by procainamide), and the drug addictions which not infrequently were initiated by legitimate medical use of the drug in question. In infancy and childhood we have had the thalidomide babies with their mismade limbs, and the very rare disasters that may follow immunizations of various sorts.

There is no question that on the balance, modern treatment of the conditions in our intrinsic group has prolonged lives and often made life more tolerable for sufferers but there is also a substantial amount on the debit side.

In earlier chapters I have given reasons why I am not hopeful of major therapeutic developments that will do something more than add piecemeal improvements to the best current treatment. The basic reason in general terms is the complexity and individuality of every human being and of every disease that is based on germinal or somatic genetic anomaly. I have said categorically and repeat the statement that because a gene can be transferred from one bacterium to another, there is not the slightest justification for hoping to replace a bad human gene with a good one. Even when we are only concerned with replacing a missing gene *product* such as insulin in diabetes, we must be aware of the many types of genetic anomaly which may give rise to such a symptom as excess sugar in the urine. I mentioned how irregular the results of treating PKU children have been and the almost daily estimations of phenylalanine in the blood that would be needed to ensure an optimal result. The application of science to treat any child with a genetic, metabolic, or immunological anomaly which is potentially lethal, at the best level possible in the light of current knowledge, will always be extravagantly expensive. It will require a small full-time team of biochemists and technicians and will subject the child to constant examinations, blood tests, and injections. In most cases that detailed control must be continued throughout life. It is the brutal fact that except in a research centre in an affluent country, and only when an individual scientist has a professional reputation to make or maintain in the relevant field, such children can only receive empirical care and will die at the first crisis in their condition. All these are rare conditions, however important may be the difficulties they raise, but they do force one to think more closely about the aims and limitations of therapy in the commoner polygenic and somatic genetic diseases and the chronic degenerative disabilities.

THE AIMS OF THERAPY

When we are dealing with basically sound individuals whose disease or disability is clearly related to the impact of the environment, the medical requirements are usually straightforward. Treatment, usually short-lasting, is required which will overcome the immediate anatomical or functional difficulty and leave the situation such that the reparative and rehabilitative capacity of the body can bring the individual back to an acceptable level of health. No patient who has overcome the initial impact and is not irretrievably damaged anatomically, should die from one of these conditions unless he is subject to some genetic weakness. Of course, there will always be the possibility of inadequate handling either from lack of facilities or lack of knowledge and of simple bad luck.

It is not so easy to be dogmatic about the treatment of intrinsic conditions many of which are characteristically chronic and progressive. I write as one who has never accepted full responsibility for medical care but has had a wide acquaintance with first-class physicians, surgeons, and paediatricians and in one way and another has kept fairly well in touch with most of the new principles of treatment as they have developed during the years since my internship in the Melbourne Hospital in 1922–3. Perhaps that is sufficient justification for trying to look for general rules in the treatment of symptoms and disease, with special reference to the place of 'drugs' now and in the future.

Perhaps because I am an immunologist I have an immense respect for maintaining the integrity of the body in the sense that ideally any surgical manipulations should aim at restoring normal anatomical and physiological conditions and that the only soluble substances (or insoluble material subject to eventual solubilization) brought into the body should be normal constituents thereof. If exceptions are to be made, good, well-thought-out reasons for their use should be clear in one's mind. I brought up a family— and occasionally vetoed the family doctor—on the principle, 'When in doubt don't do it!' When one uses non-biological substances from aspirin and barbiturates onward as drugs or uses mutilating surgery like leucotomy for a psychosis or hypophysectomy to slow the spread of breast cancer, one must be worried. Treatment of this artificial character may sometimes be unavoidable and can sometimes give most gratifying results but to use an old medical cliché, the over-all results are usually not encouraging.

It will be in line with the approach I have adopted throughout to look at the possibility of future progress in medicine, by trying to analyse the main symptoms that arise in what I have called the intrinsic diseases. In general the need is not to attempt cure—old age and the disabilities that go with it are manifestly incurable—but to ameliorate symptoms. This holds almost equally for genetic anomalies, degenerative conditions, and somatic genetic diseases. Symptomatic relief is often all that the patient asks for and in general the drug industry exists to provide that relief.

1. *Genetic abnormalities*

There are some genetic and partially genetic abnormalities which, as I mentioned in Chapter 6, can be righted by surgery to produce approximately normal anatomical relationships and a good functional result. One can mention pyloric stenosis of infants, harelip and cleft palate, and many congenital abnormalities of the heart. Where attempts must be limited to something much less than the reconstitution of normal structure as in hydrocephalus and spina bifida, the results are far less satisfactory and many would say that surgical interference is never really justifiable in these conditions.

The functional genetic anomalies can be divided operationally into four groups:

1. Conditions in which symptoms are due to the accumulation of an intermediate metabolite in excessive amounts. PKU has been discussed in some detail and there are a number of other rare genetic blocks in the metabolism of other amino acids. The only other condition that need be mentioned is galactosaemia where the dangerous substance is the second step in the body's handling of milk sugar.

Here the only approach is to remove all or most of the basic food substance from the diet. Galactosaemia is the only condition of the sort that can be satisfactorily handled. If it is recognized within the first few days of life and the infant transferred to a diet containing no lactose, i.e., without milk, a completely satisfactory result can be expected.

2. Conditions in which there is failure to produce a necessary substance. Here we must bear in mind the important reservation that the missing substance is always the end-product of a complex set of genetically controlled reactions and that the genetic block may be affecting other systems than the one in which we are interested. The classical examples are haemophilia in which one of two

clotting factors is missing, agammaglobulinaemia where the immunoglobulins are at a very low level, juvenile diabetes with insulin deficiency, and there are many rarer conditions.

In such diseases much can be done by providing 'maintenance therapy', providing artificially what the body needs but cannot make, and administering it at appropriate intervals. Haemophilia can be dealt with rather expensively by using a blood fraction from normal human blood to protect the patient when haemorrhage is inevitable as with surgery or dental extractions, and by shielding him in every way possible from injuries. It is a great over-simplification to say of either agammaglobulinaemia or juvenile diabetes, that normal gamma globulin and insulin given in proper dose cures the condition. In most they are life-saving but the continuing control of either is a difficult task, individual to each patient, and liable to end with death far earlier than in a normal individual.

3. Conditions in which a faulty cell or tissue component is produced. Sickle cell anaemia was discussed earlier along with albinism and cystic fibrosis; there are a number of other abnormalities of various sorts which produce symptoms and probably many others which do not. In these there is no logical approach to treatment.

4. I am not competent to discuss genetic anomalies of the brain and nervous system beyond what has been said earlier about schizophrenia.

2. *Degenerative diseases*

In dealing with degenerative diseases related to ageing I shall adopt the point of view raised earlier that the progressive inefficiency of function in normal ageing and many of the manifestations of premature senility, whether in one organ or system or quite general, are the result of somatic mutation and immunological responses made possible thereby. Some of the results have a considerable resemblance to those of frank genetic disease and may be listed under the same headings:

1. Here there are only a few distant analogies, sensitization to drugs like penicillin can be avoided by not using the drug and the relative delay in breaking down many drugs in old age has some slight resemblance.

2. The commonest cause of failure to produce a necessary substance is probably auto-immune disease. Admittedly there is a majority of physicians who prefer to say that there is no justification for any positive statement about the cause of the diseases that are being spoken of as auto-immune. Here, as elsewhere, I take the view that the acceptance of a disease as of unknown cause is never legitimate when reasonable hypotheses of its nature exist. The best current hypothesis is always to be replaced when a better arises, but in the interim it serves as the most appropriate guide to thought and experiment. Auto-immune attack provides the best current interpretation for those diseases showing limited destruction or atrophy of specific organs, which start at some variable adult age and continue progressively, though sometimes with remissions. The best examples from our present angle are:

a. Non-tuberculous Addison's disease of the adrenal glands where the symptoms are due to absence of the necessary and numerous adrenal hormones;

b. Pernicious anaemia which appears to result from auto-immune attack on cells of the stomach lining which produce a substance necessary to allow the absorption of the cobalt-containing vitamin B12 or cyano-cobalamin. It is something of a biological curiosity that both man and ruminants require B12 as an essential part of their metabolic machinery but cannot synthesize it. Man normally obtains his supply from meat; the cattle and sheep which provide the meat derive their B12 from the synthetic activity of micro-organisms in the rumen.

c. The late stage of thyroid disease known as Hashimoto's disease or myxoedema in which there is an increasing lack of thyroid hormone, thyroxin, with a general slowing down of metabolic activity.

Most people interested in auto-immune disease expect that late onset diabetes may soon be found to be a combination of partial genetic inadequacy and auto-immune attack but the position is not so clear as for the other three.

The treatment in all four is to provide the missing hormones or vitamin and, subject as always to the individual features of every patient, it is usually effective.

3. Conditions in which faulty or wrong components are produced by cells are not conspicuous in degenerative disease. One of the

interpretations of 'high blood pressure' (hypertensive disease) is that the hormone-like substance, renin, is produced in excessive amounts by the kidney but this is hardly analogous.

3. *Conditions based on somatic mutation*
There are a number of interesting effects of neoplastic disease (cancer in the broad sense) which can also be looked at from the operational angle in much the same way:

1. There are a number of tumours producing metabolites which in the normal individual are subject to very close control. There is a tumour called carcinoid which produces excessive amounts of serotonin, a drug-like substance which has very important local functions in the brain and in the process of inflammation. Its main symptoms are headaches and recurrent attacks of intense skin flushing. Occasionally as a medical curiosity one sees or hears of liver tumours which produce excessive amounts of some metabolite with corresponding symptoms. The usual interpretation is that this is a tumour arising from a single cell which in some way was 'locked' to a certain type of synthetic activity and transmitted this quality to all the descendant cells which make up the tumour. There is a resemblance here to the antibody-producing tumour multiple myeloma that was discussed on p. 16.

2. Since most tumours arise from a single cell, a tumour can only cause an absence of a normal body constituent by displacing and killing by its growth all or nearly all the cells of some particular functional type. A secondary deposit of cancer may destroy the pituitary gland, or leukaemia cells crowd other cells out of the bone marrow.

The part which may be played by auto-immune processes with their general resemblance to malignant or partially malignant cells has been described earlier. When a thyroid or the adrenals are destroyed by the attack of auto-immune immunocytes the resemblance to infiltration and destruction by cancer cells is probably a real one.

3. One of the most interesting features of malignant disease from the somatic genetic angle is the production of substances that are never produced by the cells from which the tumour has sprung. Lung cancer (bronchial carcinoma) is the commonest tumour of

men nowadays, for reasons that everyone knows but which cigarette manufacturers and governments regard as irrelevant to the public health. Most lung cancers kill as other cancers do with no special feature other than the extraordinary difficulty of dealing with them effectively. A small proportion, but a considerable absolute number, however, produce an abnormal product of some sort.

The most frequently recognized substances are hormones of various sorts, parathyroid hormone that raises calcium in the blood, a female sex hormone which may produce, as a symptom, enlargement of the male breast to an almost female contour and several others. There is evidence that other unusual substances requiring more subtle methods of their demonstration may also be produced. Using these findings as a basis an interesting hypothesis can be developed which is, I believe, not disproved by any available facts and which has an enlightening relevance to the general theme of this book.

Any cancer of the lung is derived from a single epithelial cell of the lining membrane of one of the larger air passages that lost its normal subservience to tissue controls. Normally such epithelial cells produce no known hormones and they are members 'in good standing' of the body community. The cancer is a clone of cellular citizens in revolt. It arose as a mutant perhaps induced, and certainly stimulated to proliferate, by local effects of cigarette smoke. As the initiating cell proliferated to a large clone, it continued to be subject to mutation and other types of genetic change. Once the break from control has been made the cell population apparently becomes more and more genetically unstable. Gross changes are indicated by irregularities in the number and structure of chromosomes and one can be certain that a variety of more subtle disorganizations also occur.

I have emphasized earlier that every body cell, and even with minor qualifications every cancer cell, carries in its nucleus the whole genetic information that was present in the zygote. Only a proportion of the DNA which carries that information is needed in a differentiated somatic cell, the rest is inhibited and inert but it is still there. With random distortions of genetic control there are bound to be occasional sub-clones developing which can both proliferate freely and produce a protein other than those appropriate to normal epithelial cells. If such a clone appeared relatively early in the development of the tumour, considerable amounts of inappropriate or abnormal protein could be produced. At least three types of such occurrence can be deduced with three different implications:

a. The aberrant protein is one normally produced by some other type of cell and therefore is native to the body and will provoke no immune response. Its existence will be undetectable *unless it is a highly active hormone.*

b. The aberrant protein is one produced by another type of body cell but one which normally is held in the cell and plays no part in the immunological give and take of the body. If such a protein is synthesized and liberated by the cancer cells an immune response against it may become evident as *an auto-immune attack* on the cells of which the protein is a normal component.

c. As a subclass of *b* there are some tumours which produce a protein which is normal in embryonic life but is not found in adult tissues.

d. The aberrant protein is so distorted from any standard pattern that it is foreign to the body and can provoke immune responses. In general, such anomalous proteins will have no significance and will only be recognized by some chance interaction in immunological tests. The exception has already been discussed in Chapter 7. When an aberrant, essentially foreign, protein becomes a standard part of the surface membrane of the cancer cell the immune response will be against the cancer itself and if the new antigen appears early enough, may cause the tumour to break down and disappear. This is the process that I have discussed under the name of immunological surveillance in Chapter 7.

Some further notes on these three types of aberrant protein may be of interest:

a. Hormones are recognizable because of the very small quantity that is needed to produce a clinically visible effect. In addition to parathormone and oestrogen the following have been reported— insulin, anti-diuretic hormone, adrenocorticotrophic hormone (ACTH), and growth hormone, the last three all being normally produced by the pituitary gland.

b. Before dealing with the auto-immune manifestations seen with some cancers it is convenient to mention the phenomenon of formation of a foetal antigen by a group of cancers of the liver and intestinal tract. The protein can be extracted from many cancers of the lower bowel, liver, or pancreas and identified by antisera made in the rabbit. What is presumably the same protein is present in gut and liver of human embryos of the first half of pregnancy.

When a cancer of the colon (lower bowel) is present it will often liberate a sufficiency of this 'carcino-embryonic antigen' (CEA) to allow its demonstration in the blood by a sensitive immunological test. With surgical removal of the tumour the blood test becomes negative unless the surgeon has failed to remove all the growth or secondary deposits are already present. Since cancer of the lower bowel is one of the commoner forms of malignant disease and CEA is produced in the large majority, there are good prospects that blood tests for this antigen in patients with obscure abdominal symptoms may become an important diagnostic aid.

This is an important example for two reasons: (1) It is the first occasion in which an antigen specific for a certain type of tumour in *all* human patients has been recognized so allowing the development of the first 'blood test for cancer' that has good scientific credentials. (2) The reappearance of a foetal antigen in a cancer arising in an adult underlines the validity of the concept that the nucleus of any body cell contains the whole content of information that was in the zygote. If one bears in mind the picture of a human life as a four-dimensional clone, the rule becomes that in principle any cell in the clone has the potentiality of doing what any other cell of the clone can do, given the right conditions.

c. Tumours are rather frequently associated with auto-immune disease: One case of special interest was observed in the Rockefeller University Hospital in New York. She was a woman with very severe rheumatoid arthritis with all the characteristic auto-antibodies, which attack the joints, in her blood. As part of a full clinical examination she was found to have a previously unsuspected lung cancer. This was surgically removed with a rapid improvement of her arthritis and the disappearance of the auto-antibodies. In about twelve months' time, however, the tumour recurred and with this fatal recurrence her rheumatoid arthritis came back in all its aspects. There was another group of cases of lung cancer under special study in London because of the occurrence of symptoms indicating interference with function of brain or nerve. In these the connection between the nervous symptoms and the lung cancer was obscure but in at least four cases there was auto-antibody against nerve cells in the blood which provides a reasonable presumption that similar cases without auto-antibody were also auto-immune in nature but involved only a cellular attack by what I called T-immunocytes earlier.

d. Only one additional comment is needed in regard to the new surface antigens on cancer cells which are called TSTA, tumour specific transplantation antigens, in the technical literature. This is to point out that it is not possible to do more than make very superficial study of this phenomenon in man. There is no lack of indirect evidence that we do have an immune surveillance mechanism but such processes can be studied in detail only when pure line strains of experimental animals are available.

These secondary effects of cancer in producing symptoms other than those due simply to its growth and invasion of adjacent tissues may throw interesting light on the genetic abnormalities to which cancer cells are subject but they offer little scope for physiologically based treatment. The only way to handle cancer is to use surgery to remove all malignant cells and when this is not possible with certainty, hope that intelligent use of X-rays will destroy the rest without more than acceptable damage to adjacent normal tissues. The rather remote possibility of obtaining tissue cultures of the patient's cancer cell clone and testing them for susceptibility to chemotherapeutic or immune attack has been discussed earlier. It has the flavour of a research project which would require quite abnormally favourable circumstances to give hope of an effective result. The demand that any new therapy should be capable of showing its superiority over current standard methods would be extremely difficult to fulfil. In this respect I should like to quote something I said on this theme of cancer treatment in 1957 which I believe still holds: '. . . treatment of cancer is one of those social problems that must be allowed to develop their own current solutions under the various pressures of advancing knowledge, of changing public opinion and of the enthusiasm or influence of advocates of this or that approach. A final solution will probably never be possible.'

This summary of the various effects of genetic, degenerative, and somatic genetic disease in relation to the possibilities of logical treatment is obviously highly pessimistic in tone. Except for continuing replacement or maintenance therapy where there is definable absence or insufficiency of a normal body component, there are very few opportunities for logical treatment that will bring conditions essentially back to normal or to a point where the reparative powers of the body can manage the return to normality. This is, of course, little more than a statement of the obvious. Most medical treatment of disease of 'intrinsic' origin must necessarily make use of synthetic drugs for dealing more or less effectively with symptoms as they arise.

THE MEDICAL USE OF 'DRUGS'

In the final section of this chapter I want to explore the use of drugs in medicine from the rather special angle that I have tried to maintain throughout this book. It is an unusual way of looking at pharmacology and is possibly somewhat naïve but I believe it throws some light on the many doubts and dissatisfactions with our modern drugs. It is well known that the Food and Drugs Administration in the United States is demanding more and more critical testing of a drug before it can be marketed, and is aiming to eliminate many older drugs and combinations of drugs whose value has never been properly established. It seems in fact that there is a growing scepticism about future developments in the use of synthetic drugs.

I know that there is a general feeling in the drug industry that discoveries that are commercially viable are becoming increasingly hard to make. I can believe it when I am told that one American firm has in recent years spent $200 million without producing a new marketable product. Pharmaceutical products are unlike almost any other article of commerce in the virtual irrelevance of their price to the consumer. A physician is logically bound to order the best possible treatment for his patient and the cost of a drug is hardly considered. It is therefore essential that if a drug manufacturer is to obtain a profit which will cover the enormous expense of research and development, he must persuade a large proportion of medical practitioners throughout the world that his preparation, (*a*) is valuable in the treatment of some *common* condition—headache, insomnia, depression, high blood pressure, hay fever, and asthma, for example—and (*b*) that it is the *best* treatment. Scientifically established capacity to remove symptoms is only one factor; acceptability to the patient and convenience for the doctor are important, so is the current fashion in prescribing, and, not as much considered as they ought to be, the unwanted side-effects that may be seen in individual patients.

It is not surprising, therefore, to be told that in America the ethical drug manufacturers spend between \$4,000 and \$5,000 per annum for each medical practitioner in the country on various forms of 'ethical' persuasion. This is just one of the facts of life in a democratic-capitalist country. It must equally be remembered, however, that virtually all the well-known modern drugs have been discovered as well as exploited in the research laboratories of the great drug firms of America, Switzerland, West Germany, and Britain.

As an outsider I am not competent to assess the virtues of any of the modern or classical drugs but I am impressed with the evidence their use has provided of the overwhelming complexity of human (or mammalian) structure which, after all, is one of the major themes of this book. To the best of my knowledge there is no clear understanding at the molecular level of how *any* drug influences cellular function in the body. Here I am not concerned with many of the anti-infectious agents where the objective is the relatively simple one of damaging some essential function of the micro-organism which is not manifested in any mammalian cells. Even in this field, one may find a potentially harmful effect on human cells. When, however, we restrict ourselves to drugs that can influence intrinsic disease we are necessarily demanding that a drug will influence one type of cell in what we believe to be a beneficial fashion but have no effect on all the other cells of the body. This is asking something which is probably impossible and to which there is no logical approach. We may speak of cell receptors which mediate drug action but these have never been defined in molecular terms. Even for a drug of such simple chemical structure as aspirin virtually nothing is known of the molecular basis of its action.

It is possible that my point about complexity may best be made by discussing briefly not a synthetic drug but one of the body's own hormones which is widely used in therapeutics, cortisone as type substance of the gluco-corticoids. In the body cortisol (or hydrocortisone) is the standard form to which cortisone can be readily converted and which can be regarded as broadly equivalent to all the synthetic and semi-synthetic drugs of the group which have been developed. There is a broad and useful interpretation of the function of cortisol initiated long ago by W. B. Cannon that it is part of the mobilization of body function to deal with a stressful situation by 'fight or flight'.

The textbook story is that appreciation of danger results in stimulation of the hypothalamic region of the brain-stem which liberates a corticotrophin-releasing factor CRF. This passes by a special, localized blood loop to the pituitary gland where it stimulates certain cells to liberate corticotrophin, also called ACTH, into the blood. ACTH is a very small protein of only thirty-nine amino acids which stimulates the cortex of both adrenal glands to liberate a complex mixture of steroid hormones, including cortisol, whose combined effect is to ready the body for stress.

When one tries to analyse the physiological effect of an increased amount of cortisol, one finds that quite an extraordinary number of bodily systems are involved. There is a mobilization of blood sugar and amino acids from accelerated protein utilization, there is destruction of lymphocytes, a variable reduction in immune responses, and a complex anti-inflammatory action which seems to involve almost all the cells and small blood vessels concerned in the inflammatory response. Finally, there is what in practical therapeutics seems to be its most important function, to prevent the damaging effect of any immune reaction involving cell surfaces. One must assume that all the cells concerned in these manifold reactions have receptors which can recognize in some sense the shape of the hydrocortisone and related molecules and in so doing provide a stimulus which sets in action an intracellular process responsible for the observed effect.

It is not always easy to see in what respect some of these reactions to cortisol are necessary or beneficial to the body's economy. The actual concentration of the hormone in the blood under different physiological circumstances may well be the critical factor and provide a clue to apparent discrepancies. Some of the effects of cortisol in large doses are clearly undesirable physiologically, for example, its effect on the immune responses. This indicates that there must be 'just right' concentrations of cortisol in the blood and (as is known to be the case) machinery to maintain such levels. It is interesting that in experiments in which antibody is being produced by fragments of spleen in a test-tube, small amounts of insulin and hydrocortisone must be present or no antibody is produced. The levels are of the order that is found in circulating blood so the phenomenon provides a useful warning against interpreting physiological function on the basis of the pharmacological effect of abnormally large doses of a natural body component.

That picture of complexity could be elaborated almost *ad infinitum*, but it is perhaps sufficient to suggest the immensely intricate flow of information in the body by which patterned molecules react with cell receptors, which are protein patterns, whose configuration is strictly determined by the cell genome, so that the cell produces other patterned molecules which in their turn react . . . in what may literally be an endlessly interlinked chain of sequences. The nervous system, and particularly the visceral or autonomic nervous system, impinges into this flow of information at many points, frequently by the liberation of active agents at the junction of the nerve-ending and the responsive cell.

The almost incredibly complex interwoven network of chemical communication that normal physiology and biochemistry has revealed, must make pharmacology seem something much less than a science. Tens of thousands of synthetic organic compounds, substances never met in the course of evolution, have been injected into animals and their effect on measurable functions of the body assessed. The approach has been almost wholly empirical, so empirical that it is quite remarkable how often a drug developed for one action has found its place in therapeutics because of what was first regarded as an unimportant side-effect. It is only a slight caricature of pharmacological investigation to say that it involves introducing such and such a substance into the animal in the hope that somewhere it will find receptors which can either be stimulated or blocked by its action. A positive effect presumably means that the substance has something in common with the known or unknown normal substances which makes use of the receptor. If the effect is sufficiently limited to one functional system the substance becomes a drug with potential usefulness in medicine.

Every detail of bodily structure has been moulded by evolution to deal with things as they are; synthetic drugs have no evolutionary meaning. A receptor for natural hormone X will have a standard recognition site adapted to X but other aspects of the receptor will probably differ according to the type of cell and the genetic constitution of the individual. If we have a series of drugs P, Q, R, which have some resemblance to X so that they can to some degree stimulate X-receptors, we should almost certainly find that P, Q, and R differed amongst themselves in at least two ways. In different individuals the range of effective concentrations of the three would probably vary widely; so would the types of side-effect observed as a result of accidental stimulation or inhibition of quite unrelated receptors.

So we find in every ethical advertisement for a drug a long list of possible side-effects, of other drugs which must not be combined with it, and of disease conditions in which the drug is contraindicated, which is a synonym for positively dangerous.

The traditional wisdom of physicians is unanimous that so long as human beings wish to be relieved of pain or of any of the other symptoms that make illness distressful, drugs must be used if they are effective and reasonably safe. It is also accepted that on occasion potentially dangerous drugs may be used to treat a dangerous situation where a large dose over a critical period may be life-saving. This holds specially for cortisol and its equivalents when they are used to calm down one of the critical situations which tend to arise in auto-immune conditions such as asthma, sympathetic ophthalmia, and rheumatoid arthritis. Nevertheless, one has a nagging certainty that we intrude into the informational network of the body at our peril. Patients can become resistant to a drug that was formerly effective, they may become sensitized so that a formerly useful drug becomes a dangerous poison, they may become dependent or addicted. It is one of the sad realities of an imperfect world that drugs are necessary at all.

We are all very much aware that the use of modern drugs has increased exponentially in recent years and it will probably continue to increase. In a calmer, less overcrowded world in which medicine could develop the single aim of maintaining and re-establishing health appropriate to age, I feel certain that we could be happy with no more than twenty to thirty synthetic drugs in our armamentarium.

Over-use of drugs on medical direction is an obvious feature of present Australian, American, or British society. There is, per-haps, a special danger in the increasing use by physicians of the psycho-active drugs that can damp down the minor distresses of interpersonal relations and so on, that are an inescapable part of life. The social problems of drug addiction and the more subtle influence of the need to use alcohol, tobacco, sedatives, tranquil-lizers, and the rest, to make intolerable situations acceptable instead of making an effort to change them, lie outside my field. But they make up an important part of the technological and social crisis of our times.

The only conclusions I can offer on the use of drugs in medicine are already implicit in what I have said. To summarize:

1. Ideally the physician's therapeutic agents should be limited to substances natural to the body.

2. The functioning human organism is far too complex to allow fully logical and predictable modification of function or of the symptoms of abnormal function, with chemical agents foreign to the body.

3. Synthetic drugs are still needed in medicine. Their use will be on an empirical basis preferably for a limited period and for a specific purpose. If prolonged use is contemplated their poten-tiality for serious harm must be carefully weighed against the benefit expected from their use.

4. The great pharmaceutical houses of the mid twentieth century may come to feature in history as examples both of the productivity of science applied to industry and of the evils inherent in the technological momentum of a competitive industrial society.

12

THE NEW OUTLOOK

In the preceding chapters I have tried to provide a picture of the difficulties of medical science in handling the problems of intrinsic disease. The picture is wholly different from what has been achieved with disease due to the impact of the environment—extrinsic illnesses due to infection, malnutrition, or trauma. There all the problems were solved in principle by the mid 1950s. There have been many interesting observations and practical achievements, particularly in regard to infectious disease, since, but 99 per cent of the advance has been based on what was known before 1955.

After working for a year on the present book I cannot avoid the conclusion that we have reached the stage in 1971 when little further advance can be expected from laboratory science in the handling of the 'intrinsic' types of disability and disease. There will always be possibilities of improvement in detail but I am specially impressed by the fact that since 1957 there has been no new thought on the handling of cancer, of old age, or of auto-immune disease. The only real novelty has been kidney transplantation which is now giving an extension of a few years of life to an increasing proportion of those receiving kidneys to replace their own. Without the introduction of any new principles an even greater contribution to survival has come from improvement in surgical skill in handling genetically based anatomical anomalies as in congenital heart disease and in applying surgery to many of the catastrophes which can involve the larger blood vessels—abdominal aneurysm, some types of cerebral haemorrhage, and even selected cases of coronary blockage. Another important development has been the steady improvement in the results of combined surgical and radiological treatment of cancer. This holds for most of the common sites, with primary lung cancer the only important exception, and it is probably here that there has been the greatest increase in man-years of survival during the last decade.

Unfortunately the other feature of the decade has been the rising death-rates from lung cancer, from coronary disease, from road accidents, and from the direct and indirect effects of alcoholism and drug addiction. The increased loss of man-years here must far exceed the gain from improved surgery of cancer and genetic disabilities. The real problem of today is to find some means of diminishing the incidence of these diseases of civilization. To discuss that lies outside my theme but it remains the most urgent and difficult challenge in medicine. Nothing from the laboratories seems to have any relevance to such matters.

ARE WE WAITING FOR THE END?

All this is unhappy stuff for someone to be writing who thoroughly enjoyed a professional career in laboratory research on infectious disease and immunology. None of my juniors seems to be worried as I am, that the contribution of laboratory science to medicine has virtually come to an end. The biomedical sciences all continue to provide fascinating employment for those active in research, and sometimes enthralling reading for those like me who are no longer at the bench but can still appreciate a fine piece of work. But the detail of an RNA phage's chemical structure, the place of cyclostomes in the evolution of immunity or the production of antibody in test-tubes are typical of today's topics in biological research. Almost none of modern basic research in the medical sciences has any direct or indirect bearing on the prevention of disease or on the improvement of the medical care.

A more widely based and disturbing opinion about the laboratory sciences themselves quite apart from their bearing on medicine has been voiced by two near contemporaries of mine, Gunther Stent and Niels Jerne, both of them distinguished experimentalists. They feel that both biological and physical science may have passed the era of the great discoveries. I have to agree with them and can quote a statement I made elsewhere, that future historians may speak of an age of scientific discovery that started with Galileo in 1586 and ended something less than four hundred years later. If one looks at the volume of competent scientific work being produced in all fields in 1971, that statement may seem utter nonsense. There is more than ever before and the general technical competence with which the experimental work has been done is higher than ever. But the new discovery when it comes usually has an air of triviality for any one not actually working in the field in which it has been made. Compared to the great days of the 1930s for particle physics or the 1950s for molecular biology, the late 1960s were not very productive. It is significant that the major new discoveries were observational rather than experimental and depended on the availability of very advanced technological equipment. Probably the most important recent discovery has been the direct evidence of ocean floor spreading and continental drift, obtained by the study of cores from the deep ocean bed.

Until oceanographers could make use of the equipment and the knowledge developed for oil drilling on the continental shelf and for the military use of submarines, the bottom of the ocean was almost as inaccessible as the edges of the universe.

In the world of astronomy, radar can explore further than the great optical telescopes and the great discoveries of the 1960s, quasars and pulsars, derive from the ultra-sophisticated 'dishes' of the radio-astronomers used virtually to their limit of resolution. There is no doubt that in due course they will reveal more about the history of the universe. As at present the physical information about them seems to be consistent with several alternative and mutually incompatible theories of their significance in the cosmological picture.

In the fundamental biology the last major discovery was the completion of the genetic code.

I believe the analogy that Niels Jerne drew with the history of geographic discovery is a valid one. We can all have an immensely detailed interest in the little area of the world that we move in but for the rest we are satisfied when we have an approximate picture of the distribution of the continents and oceans on the globe and find it familiar and easy to use an atlas to check where some newsworthy catastrophe has occurred. There have been good atlases since the middle of the nineteenth century. What has been done since then has been to fill in the detail and keep the picture up to date.

I believe that in all the major sciences the general picture has been competently and in broad outline completely delineated by 1970. The task now is to fill in the detail and where we are dealing with observational sciences like meteorology or ecology keep the picture up to date. In many ways I should like to believe that I am as wrong as those scientists who said the same about physics in the early 1890s. It has been exciting to watch the great discoveries in the sciences emerge during the last fifty years and one would like the next generation to have some of the same pleasure. But everything must come to an end and I think that I can already see signs that scientists are recognizing this and modifying their activities accordingly. Ecology and ethology, two predominantly observational sciences now hold pride of place in biology because of their rather direct bearing on contemporary human problems. Environmental pollution has suddenly brought words like ecology, ecosystem, and biosphere into the common vocabulary. The fashionable approach to human conflict is to seek enlightenment from animal behaviour via the ethologists, Lorenz, Tinbergen, and Washburn, for example, or their popular interpreters, Ardrey, Desmond Morris, Koestler, and, at a lower level, perhaps I could claim to join them. Environmental studies are calling for the most advanced techniques, with satellite photography in the infra-red, likely to become the key approach to large-scale work. The eruption of human conflict with violence into the campus has brought enormous academic interest in aggression, animal and human.

In the past, public interest in science was almost wholly limited to the bearing of new discoveries on human affairs and especially to the possibility that some of these results could be applied to human benefit—or to avoid begging an important question—for the satisfaction of human needs or desires. The human and social situation of the scientists as a group within the community provoked very little interest when the number of scientists was insignificantly small. This is no longer the case. Scientific research and development over-all employs a substantial proportion of the professional workers in any advanced country, and when one adds teachers of science and those in the growing industries that supply instruments, reagents, etc., for scientific work, it may amount to 1 per cent or more of the work force and up to 5 per cent of university graduates and other professionals.

THE FUTURE OF SCIENCE IN RELATION TO SOCIETY

In discussing the future of science I believe that our starting point in 1971 must be with the existing body of scientists and the larger number of young people in training for a scientific career. This will, initially at least, take me rather a long way from my primary topic but it is an essential aspect of today's approach to put primary emphasis on the human side of social problems.

Probably the greatest change in social pattern of the last seventy years has been the reduction of the proportion of people employed in agriculture and stock-raising from 50 to 10 per cent or less in advanced Western countries. One man on the land can feed ten or more in the cities. The surplus from the country has been absorbed into secondary and tertiary industry in the towns. The next step in the same direction will clearly be a progressive increase in productivity per man-hour in secondary industry as a result of automation and computer-based management. Workers displaced will, hopefully, be employed by the various tertiary industries concerned with finance, administration, including government service, health care, and other types of personal service to the individual, education, and scientific research.

The most important relevant feature in the political background against which these changes are taking place, will probably be the efforts to deal with three critical situations. I can foresee serious attempts being made (a) to limit and lower population levels in all countries; (b) to disarm, especially in nuclear weapons; and (c) to slow down technological innovation until the problems of environmental deterioration are caught up with. I would go further and say, as I have done in another book, that unless all three can be accomplished, civilization will vanish within a hundred years, and perhaps much sooner.

The most important short-term result of any such action will undoubtedly be unemployment. As in everything, America provides the pattern of what comes next. There is already an unemployment problem despite the large numbers of men in the armed services and the millions of young people of working age who are kept off the labour market by their continuing education in universities or other institutions of tertiary education. If disarmament were accepted the situation would become much more difficult, and if unemployment were avoided by the necessary expansion of secondary industry, matters might be even worse. Every country except perhaps Australia, has too many people and too little space. To provide the average citizen throughout the world with what he desires by the full application of modern technology and manpower on the American pattern would un-doubtedly mean an accelerating and irreversible deterioration of the environment. The problems are not solved by expanding secondary industry.

Until world population trends are reversed and numbers brought down to a tolerable level the need will be to find acceptable occupation that gives a sense of social usefulness for the increasing numbers of people not needed in primary or secondary industry. Amongst them will be many scientifically trained people in the upper intelligence brackets. It will be a pre-emptive requirement of the immediate future and for as long as civilization may survive, that high-level scholarly activities in science should continue and expand. For very similar reasons a social structure must be developed which will allow a great increase in the numbers of people doing skilled manipulative work both in the fine arts and in personal craftsmanship at various levels.

What must be thought of particularly is that scientific work should be such as will not lead to further pollution of the environ-ment nor foster war or other forms of human conflict. On the positive side it must provide opportunity for achievement and for recognition of success of much the same quality as has been traditional in the scientific community. It interests me very much that to a large extent this is how science and technology is at present advancing.

In the physical-technical field the desirable advances are in machines to facilitate communication and the processing of in-formation. Such apparatus uses little raw material, does not con-taminate the environment during its functioning and uses much skilled professional and technical labour. The range would include all types of electronic data-processing machines, including their applications to education and research, advanced telecommunica-tions including colour television, videophones, and satellite com-munications. In all these, the requirement is the application of known principles and techniques at a very high level of technical skill and accuracy.

The second major need for at least the immediate future is the development of measures to counter pollution and environmental deterioration and to rehabilitate the regions that have been harmed. The importance of this is already recognized by most governments with Sweden and America in the lead. Its significance can hardly be over-estimated as a source of socially useful employment in the inevitable period of gross overpopulation and potential unemployment in front of us.

FUTURE OF THE BIOLOGICAL SCIENCES

In our proper sphere of the biological and medical sciences we can assume first that the population explosion is fairly rapidly checked and reversed. If this does not happen, food production and sewage disposal could well become the main interest of most biologists. If things turn out more satisfactorily, I believe that biological research can provide gratifying occupation for as many people as have the necessary training, competence, and motivation. For reasons I have tried to express in earlier chapters I do not expect conventional benefits to medicine or technology from biological research to be common in the future. If they should arise they may be accepted as bonuses but need not be sought.

Scholarly biological research in the future will, as now, be broadly divisible into laboratory studies and ecological work. The latter will probably always include a substantial amount of applied research in the agricultural and veterinary fields and a greater likelihood that scholarly work will provide spin-off of practical significance.

1. *Laboratory research*

In Chapter 11 the complexity of the mammalian body was blamed for the ineffectiveness of our approach to the problems of genetic disease, senescence, cancer, etc. Yet in the present context, complexity is a positive advantage. There is no stage in biological research on a chosen topic when that topic will be exhausted. To take perhaps the most closely studied molecule in the mammalian body, haemoglobin, there is still much to be done in following the process by which it is synthesized in reticulocytes, and the mechanism by which three successive types ε, γ, and β chains are produced during embryonic development. An almost infinite range of organisms remain to be examined for information on the evolution of haemoglobin structure and of the function of the primordial chains. There is even the intriguing problem of the ice-fish which manage without haemoglobin—the only vertebrates to do so. Every other biological topic has these two additional dimensions, as it were, of development in the individual and of evolutionary history and significance.

In my own field of immunology this possibility of limitless elaboration still with the capacity to provoke enthusiastic interest can be seen very clearly at the present time in the analysis of amino acid sequences in the immunoglobulin chains. This work has implications still to be clarified for the nature of the antibody combining site, the genetic mechanism by which diversity of immune pattern is generated, and the evolutionary history of the genes whose duplications have made the complex immunoglobulins possible. Before that programme has gone very far I expect it to impinge strongly on the question of cell membrane structure and provoke another dozen fascinating problems. Here we have a programme immensely attractive to a scholar and at this moment occupying some of the best brains in biological research, Porter, Putnam, Kabat, Edelman, Edman, and many others. It is being carried out in the major medical research centres of the world— and it has no more bearing on the prevention or cure of disease than the study of quasars or 'black holes' in galactic centres. It is a paradigm of the research of the future.

There are doubtless a thousand or more aspects of mammalian function—thereby qualifying as medical research!—which could each grow into an equivalent programme of laboratory work but I shall say only a word or two about a topic that has already been discussed in Chapter 3. The techniques developed by Beatrice Mintz for fusing two mouse blastocysts to produce a single viable mouse has opened a basically new approach to the analysis of differentiation and cell migrations in the embryo. It is something which in due course could be applied to any substance or function in which two pure line strains of the same species of experimental animal were known to differ. In the process many new lines of research will arise. We have already a growing number of ways by which cells can be labelled and their movement and progeny identified. There is virtually no limit to the use of such techniques in this field of laboratory research into the nature of cellular differentiation and organ building. This is the wave of the future in biology but one must not expect from it either a complete understanding of the mechanics of development or any significant applications to practical affairs. What can be predicted with some certainty is that the fused-blastocyst technique of Mintz is only the first of many experimental *models*. With each of them, some new phase of development will become available for study and new provisional generalizations become possible.

2. *Ecological studies*

In the ecological field the opportunities are even greater for endlessly satisfying work. Every country can provide countless ecosystems any one of which offers material for productive study. It is one of the virtues of ecology that almost every good investigation must be an inter disciplinary one involving scientists from a dozen or more fields. As examples I shall mention only two, both, for obvious reasons, Australian.

In western Australia there are great tracts of arid country, irregularly visited by rain in which a wide variety of marsupials, frogs, spiders, and insects make a living. For most of the year the environment is very dry and hot. Main and Waring for the last fifteen years have been asking how those four groups of animals obtain and retain their body water. They are combining physiological experiments in the laboratory with field studies and have found some extraordinary capacities. There is a wallaby on some of the off-shore islands which survives for months on a diet of sun-dried grass and seawater!

In any ecological study there are always other dimensions in which the central phenomenon of interest can be explored. Often, as in Main's studies, laboratory work with the species is required; evolutionary problems come into the picture and always call for knowledge of at least the Pleistocene and Recent geology of the area. Nearly always, too, there is the necessity to follow the phenomenon as it changes with season and under the impact of drought, flood, or human interference.

A distinguished scholar in cytological genetics in Melbourne is interested in the relationship of chromosome patterns in grasshoppers to their ecology. His domain of study covers much of south-eastern Australia and very little of the original native grasses remain in the settled areas. In nearly every little country town, however, there is an enclosure of a few acres which has neither been grazed nor cultivated for a hundred years. It is the local cemetery fenced off when the town first established its identity and always with a large neglected area carrying its native grass. For certain groups of grasshoppers, Professor X assured me, the only way to establish the original distribution of karyotypes in southern New South Wales and Victoria, is to collect the insects exclusively in cemeteries!

There is an obvious moral in that story. In a country like Australia still being opened up for cultivation in places, in other parts, over-exploited in the past and now deserted, and irregularly subject to drought or flood, plant and animal populations are constantly changing. Continuing surveys in 'real time' by teams of systematists and ecologists could be relied on to provide a never-ending source of illuminating material from which a good scientist would gain both satisfaction and prestige among his peers.

3. *Clinical research*

Finally we come back to medicine and here again there seems to be no problem in finding satisfying careers for those who wish to see science applied to the limit in keeping people alive or, more desirably in ensuring complete and rapid rehabilitation after illness. It does not seem likely that wholly new principles of treatment will emerge but there was probably never an occasion when an enthusiastic group combining clinical research and patient care in a study of some type of illness, failed to get better results than the average for their hospital or community. Computer-aided diagnosis is certainly on the horizon and holds out some interesting possibilities for new types of epidemiological study. The whole basis of disease classification within the group of 'intrinsic' conditions could well change completely and I should expect a good computer analysis of symptoms and an adequate list of physical signs and blood concentration of relevant metabolites in relations to age will turn out to be enlightening to the gerontologist.

The world may be approaching a stage when population increase, war, pollution, and exhaustion of resources will produce a nightmare situation that ends in chaos. If good sense and good luck give us an affluent peaceful era with population at least stabilized, I see no reason why biological and medical research should not be more active and satisfying in the future than ever in the past. But we shall have to forego that special place we used to claim amongst scholars that there was special virtue in our work because of its potentiality for saving life.

Once a certain stage of intellectual sophistication has been reached there is almost always a need to feel satisfaction with what one does with one's life. Each of us with, I suspect, varying degrees of insight and honesty, will be liable to ascribe this satisfaction to its compatibility with some accepted value. The prevention of disease and the prolongation of life have been universally accepted by modern communities as of unequivocal value. It has been easy to apply that value to what we were doing in the laboratories. As the phrase goes, it gave meaning to our lives.

When we can no longer accept that particular relevance, it becomes more difficult to find an answer for the man who asks where a biological scientist looking squarely at the human situation can find meaning in life. My own answer, which I have expanded in another book, will be regarded as unacceptably élitist by many but it is the best I can find. It is that the only virtue of an affluent society has always been that it provides a means by which the men and women who have the capacity and the drive to do something really well can find opportunity to do it and gain satisfaction, both in the achievement and in the recognition and reward it brings.

I found immense gratification all through my forty years of laboratory research, but the background attitude progressively changed from a naïve concern for doing good, through various phases of doubt and cynicism, to a conviction that scholarly work in science must be equated not only with scholarly work in the humanities but also with the creative ability of artist, writer, or composer, and in fact with any type of achievement that can be rated by competent judges as outstandingly good.

INDEX

Where the page number is shown in **bold** type this normally indicates a main discussion of the indexed subject.